M000091917

Praise for Dad Named Me Robert

This is a compelling and fascinating story of the life of Robert, who has schizophrenia. It is uniquely written by his mother who specializes in the brain basis of mental illnesses. Over more than thirty years, I have been awed at the advocacy and care that Joan and her family provided for Robert.

Throughout Joan's faculty career, she has helped teachers, nurses, policemen, other professionals, and families understand the brain basis of mental illness. Joan gives an inside story of what it's really like to live with a son who has schizophrenia.

Karyl Rickard, PhD, RDN
Professor Emeritus of Nutrition and Dietetics
Indiana University School of Health and Human Sciences
Indianapolis, IN

Marvelous! I laughed and cried all the way through the book. So many poignant chapters. Love it! Joan shares the practical aspects of daily care and all the research, with wisdom more than most know. Joan and her family are a rare family who pull together and make more than 30 years with schizophrenia work for them and for Robert's care. It's their love and faithfulness that made this work.

Ann Schwab, Retired Mental Health Nurse

Dad Named Me
Robert

Let's Talk About Mental Illness

JOAN ESTERLINE LAFUZE, PH.D.

Joan Esterline Lafuze

March 2021

First Printing

Copyright 2020 ©Joan Esterline Lafuze, Ph.D.

ISBN: 978-1-64184-327-0 (Hardcover)
ISBN: 978-1-64184-328-7 (Paperback)
ISBN: 978-1-64184-329-4 (eBook)

Publisher
Sojourn Publishing, LLC
Sedona, AZ

Printed in the United States of America

Mom, I know that Dad gave me my name, Robert,
but Mom, what I really want to ask is how
Dad knew that was the name God wanted for me?

Dedication

Robert, this book is dedicated to you.
You opened a wonderful, wide world of friendship and
understanding that without you we would not have known.
Many times, we've been told how fortunate you were to
have us as your family. May this story tell the world that our
family was truly fortunate to have had *you.*

In your honor, all book proceeds will support the Indiana
University Foundation's Robert Lawrence Lafuze Scholars
Fund, which assists pre-medical students at Indiana
University East.

Table of Contents

Acknowledgements

I hesitate to acknowledge any person by name in expressing my gratitude, for all of you have truly blessed our lives. Our family has extended far beyond the bounds of biology. Each of you, whether family or friend, has had a role in the writing of this book. I thank **you**.

I acknowledge all of Ralph's and my family members. You have been so much a part of Robert's life. He loved each one of you dearly. I mention, especially, the families of my sisters, Jan and Mary, the families of Ralph's sisters, Janice and Rosemary, and the families of my daughters, Jeannette, Leanne, Mary, and Jan Adams.

There have been so many more physicians from different specialties who have cared for Robert and for our family than I could ever name. I am truly grateful to each one of you. Here I acknowledge by name seven psychiatrists and one family-practice physician who have provided special care and support since Robert's psychotic break in 1981. Thank you, Dr. Andy Chambers, Dr. John Delaney, Dr. Stephen Dunlop, Dr. Jeffrey Kellams, Dr. Jeffrey Kons, Dr. Michael Metrick, Dr. Alan Schmetzer, and Dr. Anantha Shekhar.

This book would not have been written without the very practical assistance of The Tom Bird Organization, Denise Cassino, Sue McFadden, and Janice Wilkins.

Foreword

When Joan emailed me to ask if I could write a foreword to her
book about Robert, there was no way I could deny her request.
That is not because, as she says in the book, I have researched
the stigma of mental illness. Yes, it is true that I stumbled into
a research concern with stigma as I tried to understand how
individuals face crisis. Rather, it was because Joan is one of
the kindest people I have ever encountered in my life. This was
a fact that had amazed me as I learned of the struggles in her
own life, with her children, her career, and with the medical
system. She had every reason to be angry, to be nasty, and
to be closed off, given the hand she had been dealt. Yet, she
radiated calm, wisdom, and a sweetness that remains indelible
in my mind to this day.

I don't exactly recall how I met Joan, whether it was through
FACET (Faculty Colloquium for Excellence in Teaching),
Indiana University's teaching award and community network
of professors working to improve higher education, or through
the NIMH R24 grant that I received to bring together Indiana
researchers working on issues focused on serious mental illness.
It matters little. In both venues, Joan was a strong voice of
commitment and concern, always with a hopeful view of change
that we could make things happen. She came with unique
insight that translated into research and then into action. She
was among the first to ask (and research) how the clergy saw
people with mental illness in their congregations, and how they
responded to them. The answer was startling. They didn't see

them at all. That is, the clergy reported a welcoming attitude but indicated that they had no individuals with serious mental illness among their congregations. What the clergy did not understand was that religion has not always been kind to those with mental illness, in early times seeing them as possessed by the devil. What the clergy did not understand was that this history had taken its toll. Despite the commonly stated statistic that one in four people in the US will experience at least one episode of mental health problems in their lives, that history silenced the people in their churches for fear of stigma and the exclusion that it typically brings.

Joan writes pointedly and poignantly about the deadly consequences of prejudice and discrimination attached to mental illness. Whether describing the inability of strangers to see Robert's future (public stigma), or the prejudices built into the treatment of mental illness (structural stigma), her words strike at the heart of the fundamental walls that individuals, families, providers, and communities face. But to her great credit, and with amazing humility, she describes her battles to overcome these cultural and institutional obstacles. She clarifies for us both the hurdles to jump and the ways to jump them. Her mantra (We are not here to blame. We are here to solve problems.) captures her spirit so well. And, Joan did this with a grace that few of us can muster.

I know this because Joan was not only a key figure in my research history but also in my personal history. I did not get into sociology to save the world; I did not get into studying how people face challenges to help "the mentally ill"; and I did not get into studying mental illness because I faced a personal crisis. Nevertheless, at forty-four, well into my research agenda, I found myself the mother of a child who was not neurotypical. While my son does not face the disabling symptoms that Robert did, Joan's experiences resonated strongly with me as I think back to navigating the diagnoses, the lack of appropriate services in schools and pediatrician offices, and the endless worry about stigma. More importantly, I had the exceptional good fortune of knowing Joan, having Joan as an expert in the biological side of mental health differences, and as a friend who would take my panicked calls. I recall reading the summary of a scientific paper that showed that children with ADHD who had taken stimulant medication had more "white matter" in their brains after seven years compared to similarly diagnosed children who had not taken medication. Riddled with concern and guilt over having put my child on various forms of Ritalin and buoyed by these findings, I called Joan in a fury of hope. Knowing just enough (from Joan) about the biology of mental illness to be dangerous, I asked: "So, since the white matter is related to connections across brain regions, does this mean that we can expect better functioning and outcomes?" Joan, in her quiet and determined way, went on to explain that we really didn't know what those findings meant but that we could be hopeful. Not exactly the answer I was hoping for; but nevertheless, I was comforted by Joan's endless optimism.

And, as she details in the book, Joan is right. Things are not as bad as they once were. We have seen an acknowledgement of the biological roots of mental illness, and with it, an acceptance by the public of this information. In our own National Stigma Studies, we describe how the public's endorsement of the neurobiology of mental illnesses has improved over the last two decades, now reaching levels over 85 percent. But Joan is also right, we are not there yet. The adoption of a medical view of mental illness does not translate into the public endorsing less stigma. There is more there. There is more underneath stigma and more to be done to fight stigma. Her insights on the use or misuse of the term "behavioral health" are strikingly on target. While at a loss for a better option, no one embraces the notion of "behavioral" health. Many researchers don't like it; it does not decrease stigma; and the public doesn't know what it means. Even those of us who have not faced the severity of the situation that Robert, Joan and her family faced, we have all pushed up against the limits of the medical and social service systems and not successfully pushed them forward. As a professor at IU, every week I struggle with recommendations for student and parents who call me for help finding care. As a parent, I struggle to this day with finding providers during the transition between childhood and adulthood, with services that are not pharmacological to address problems in living, and with knowing that my child will have a shot at a fulfilling life. As a researcher, I struggle with NIMH's decision in the 1990s to ignore stigma as part of its portfolio and with the low funding amounts for mental illness that do not match its prevalence, the unmet treatment needs, and the concern for going beyond symptom reduction.

Yet, it is Joan's spirit that brings me to end on the enormous strides we have made. Despite some of the factors mentioned above, the turn of the 21st century saw a resurgence in stigma research which, for whatever reason, also has caught fire among the public. We see more individuals disclosing their mental health struggles without shame or excuse. We see a younger generation who embrace difference in a way that we have not seen before, and we see institutions trying to figure out solutions. These new and promising developments, where we find ourselves now, represent battles that have been hard fought, especially by people like Joan and by the bright light that was her son, Robert. Thank you, Joan. Thank you, Robert.

Bernice Pescosolido, Ph.D.
Distinguished Professor of Sociology at
Indiana University, Bloomington

Chapter 1

The Promise

I solated! Alone and very, very sad. How had I ended up here? I might as well have been a thousand miles from home and the people who knew me best. I looked at the clock on the wall of the tiny room that felt like a prison cell.

I glanced at the clock on the wall and heard its annoying tick, tick, tick. Sometimes I could not hear it at all because of the commotion, clatter and chatter, up and down the hall outside the door to my prison room. Now in the middle of the night the clock and its tick only reminded me of my longing for the touch of a loving hand and a warm human body stretched out beside me.

I waited for what seemed like a half hour to pass before I looked again at the ugly clock. How could it be that its long hand betrayed that only ten long minutes had passed? I should have known by the number of ticks, but I had blocked those from my lonely world.

I struggled to remind myself that my "guards" were kind and loving professionals who were so busy doing their job that they had forgotten I was wide awake in Room 10. Most of the other women were sleeping. I had refused sedation because the discomfort in my tummy was far better than the dizzying feeling of a world spinning out of control, further and further away. Refusing the medications was an easy choice for me.

In some ways, the sense of total isolation was worse in the daytime when there was clatter, chatter, and the noise of equipment moving past Room 10. That small world was oblivious to the wide-awake woman who felt all alone there. The least offensive times were evenings. The world outside Room 10 calmed down because there was less hustle and bustle. Personnel no longer strained their voices to be heard above the noise of the day.

One evening the excitement across the hall broke the monotony of my confinement. A woman in a room there was not dilating appropriately. Her doctor decided that perhaps the medication to sedate her was slowing the progress of her labor. I heard him instruct the nurse, whose last name was Smith, to discontinue the sedatives. The doctor told her he was leaving to attend a family birthday celebration and gave her the number of the family member who was having the party.

Memory reminds me that there were no cell phones way back then. No longer under the effects of sedation, the woman began to have stronger and stronger contractions. The nurse also checked and saw that she was dilating. I heard her call to assistants to see whether the doctor was still in the building. I was certain she was hoping that he had dawdled in the doctor's changing room. I heard the assistant come back with the announcement that she had called the woman at the front desk who had told her the doctor had left the building five minutes before.

The nurse was anxious. I could hear it in her voice. "Call this number he gave me and tell whoever answers to meet him and keep him in the car so he can turn around and come back to deliver this baby!" After fifteen minutes or so I heard the nurse say, "Help me wheel this mom to the delivery room. She cannot wait any longer."

The scene I remember after that was as follows: I saw the doctor, shirtless, tying his scrubs and running past my door. I heard the nurse cry out, "Thank God you're here!" Then I heard a baby cry and the doctor shout, "Smith, you deliver yours, and I'll deliver mine!"

I share this incident with you because it is the one memory of my experience in Room 10 that broke the pattern of loneliness. Another reason is because it is a memory that has lived on in my life. To this day, when I meet a deadline just in time, I remember with a smile, "Smith, you deliver yours, and I'll deliver mine."

It was much different this time than with my first baby girl, Jeannette. With her, my first signs of labor were contractions that grabbed my attention shortly after dinner the night before. My husband, Ralph, and I went into the hospital in the middle of the night, and she was born in the morning with a doctor and a room full of nurses and attendants who were eager to watch this "weird woman" who was wide awake while she was having this baby.

Before Jeannette was born, Ralph and I had attended Lamaze classes at Saint Vincent Hospital in Indianapolis. This program gave couples the option of staying together during the entire labor process. Husbands were trained to coach their wives to breathe with the contractions right up to the time of delivery which, at that time, was still in a separate delivery room. My goodness! How times have changed from then to now!

Ralph had been a lawyer with his uncle in a practice in downtown Indianapolis. He moved us to Richmond, Indiana when I was around seven months pregnant with Jeannette, because he wanted to be more a part of his children's lives than he pictured was possible in a large downtown firm. When we relocated, we found that the hospital was traditional. Fathers were permitted neither in the labor nor delivery rooms. Memory reminds me that the "germ" theory thrived in most hospitals in the early 1960s, and women in labor were heavily sedated so that the separation from family members did not matter much anyway.

Fifteen months after Jeannette was born, I was about to deliver again. This baby girl was different. She was very small.

I knew approximately when she was conceived and had only had a few periods in between because I had nursed Jeannette. I learned to smile in response to well-meaning doctors and nurses whose repeated message was, "Surely you counted wrong."

This time when the contractions began and Ralph and I went to the hospital, I was given medication to stop the contractions. The doctor explained that the baby was too small to survive. He assured me that if the contractions were true labor, they would overcome the medication, and I would deliver the baby. The nurse told me that it was not just the baby's small size, but the heart rate was in the range of a baby girl. Ralph and I practiced "division of labor." I bore the babies and he named them. This second daughter, he named Kathryn Jane.

Memory reminds me that in 1963 there was no ultrasound. There was no way to know how far a woman was into a pregnancy. There was no easy way to know the sex of her baby.

The obstetrician predicted well. At about 2:00 a.m. on Friday, June 21, I found myself in that same delivery room. I saw the look of concern on the obstetrician's face as he delivered a baby boy who did not make a sound. He handed the baby off to the nurse with instruction to suction him immediately while he attended to me. I heard the baby whimper. They rushed him out of the room to an incubator and the obstetrician went to tell Ralph what he did not tell me. He believed that our newborn son would not survive.

I saw the worried look on Ralph's face but all I could say was, "I think that Kathryn Jane is not going to work well." Ralph said without hesitation, "His name is Robert Lawrence Lafuze." I was surprised by the fact that this name was entirely different from any that he had mentioned if Jeannette had been a boy. Later, the experience led Ralph to a decision that when I was pregnant the next time, he would not name the baby before he saw it.

Robert was, I believe, full term. He had eyelashes and fingernails. He weighed three pounds and fourteen ounces with a normal-sized head. His body, arms, and his legs were very small. I have seen pictures of malnourished children from third world countries who have normal-sized heads, but very small bodies, arms, and legs that remind me of Robert as a newborn.

Mother Lafuze, Ralph's mother, visited us in the hospital. As we watched through the window, the nurse took Robert out of the incubator to change his diaper. I saw and heard Mother Lafuze gasp as she gazed on Robert's tiny little limbs. She visited because I would leave after a few days, and only Ralph and I could visit at that point. Robert was considered "premature" in those days. Today he would be in what is called a NICU or Neonatal Intensive Care Unit, which meets the needs of not only premature babies, but also those of newborns with unique health issues.

I had not held Robert yet. Although I intended to nurse him and used the pump to keep a milk supply for him, he was not given breast milk. At that time, formula was considered more appropriate because babies gained weight faster on it. I believed differently because I had taken immunology courses in school.

I remember standing at that window begging Robert to breathe. *Breathe, baby, breathe, and I will never forget how grateful I will be.* It is a promise I kept for fifty-five years, eight months and nine days when his care passed from me to both of his Fathers in Heaven.

Chapter 2

We Will Take Him Home
and Love Him

Robert had challenges that many do not, but he also had many successes.

Robert's Early Bonding with Ralph

One early serious challenge began when he was six months old. He had repeated ear infections. When Jeannette cried in the night, I got up, cared for her, and when I crawled back into bed, Ralph would say sleepily, "Have you been up?" When Robert cried, Ralph was out of bed and down the hall to his room. The next morning, I would find Ralph lying asleep on the floor with Robert, a little bundle of humanity, cuddled on Ralph's chest with the offending ear down to receive the warmth from his father's body. The memory is good.

Our First Trip to Riley

I recall one morning when Robert was ill. His temperature on the mercury thermometer (it was the only kind of thermometer we had back then) registered 100°. That reading created a dilemma for me because it was borderline. When an infant had a temperature over 102°, I always called the doctor's office.

The pediatrician told me to watch Robert closer than Jeannette because he was so small that he could dehydrate faster, especially with a fever.

I checked him often during the morning. In the early afternoon, he was hot to the touch. When I took his temperature, the mercury went to the top of the column. I must have grabbed Jeannette, but all I remember is running the three blocks south to the pediatrician's office with Robert clutched in my arms.

The doctor treated him on the spot to bring the fever down and told me to take him to the hospital immediately. He would call with orders. A neighbor must have taken us to the hospital. I don't remember the details of that, but I remember the comment of the nurse in pediatrics. We must have arrived before the doctor sent orders, or he simply gave her the orders with no explanation. When I arrived at the pediatric unit with Robert, she asked about his feeding schedule. Before I could explain that I was breastfeeding him on demand, she said, "Of course we will feed him more often than you are."

I remember just nodding. It was not a time to argue, but the pediatrician must have explained the entire story to her later. I remember thinking how sad it was that some babies they saw probably were malnourished. I know that the doctor must have explained that Robert was not one of them. Although she never apologized, she leaned over backwards to be friendly, treat me kindly, and with respect.

The pediatrician talked to me while Robert was in the hospital about our taking him to Riley Hospital at the Medical Center in Indianapolis for evaluation. Although he was full term, in those days he was classified as premature. When his weight did not catch up with that of most babies who were premature, his diagnosis changed to "failure to thrive." In addition, the doctor was concerned that Robert's head was disproportionately large for his body. That fact raised a question of the possibility of hydrocephalus.

When we took Robert to Riley Hospital the doctors there told us he would need to be admitted for extensive evaluation.

We had to leave him there. It was a long, silent, two-hour trip home. I was limited in the number of times I could visit him because we only had one car. Visits depended on my ability to find transportation from our home in Richmond to Riley Hospital in Indianapolis and childcare for Jeannette. Both of those had to align with visiting hours at Riley.

I was not allowed to hold him even though I was breast-feeding him. During those visits my eyes would fill with tears and my breasts with milk. It was a difficult time for us all. At the end of the several weeks he was at Riley, the doctor talked with us about having them keep him there.

They had ruled out hydrocephalus but still could not account for his enlarged head. Ralph asked whether he could simply have a normal-sized head on a small body. The doctor looked at him as if he were joking. Ralph was not. As the doctor talked on and on Ralph said, "I don't hear a plan here. Is there one?" The doctor looked at us and said, "You are foolish to have hope for this child." I was stunned, but I heard my husband say, "Then we will take him home and we will love him." And so, we did.

Chapter 3

My Acorn in the Meadow

Despite the medical concerns, Robert was an easy baby. Two of his three sisters had colic, but Robert slept and ate on schedule. He seemed happy to be alive. When he was six months old, frequent earaches caused him to cry out in pain in the night.

Because his head was large for his body and because his muscles failed to develop normally, he was unable to sit up, stand up, roll over, or crawl on schedule. In fact, only one of his sisters crawled and climbed as a baby. There was an emphasis in those days related to crawling and reading ability. It had something to do with development of eye-hand coordination. We smiled as the kids grew up. All became excellent readers, but the one least interested in reading was the one who crawled.

Of greater concern was the delay in walking. None of the four were walking at a year, but Robert's sisters walked at thirteen, sixteen and seventeen months. When Robert was not walking at eighteen months the pediatrician ordered X-rays that showed his spine had not closed fully. The pediatrician told me that he didn't expect him to walk or toilet train. However, when he was two and a half years old, he stood up one afternoon and walked. He toilet-trained easily when he was three. We were on a roll!

Just about the time that Robert walked I figured out that I was pregnant with Leanne. Please remember this was before pregnancy tests. I made an appointment with the obstetrician who had delivered both Jeannette and Robert.

When I went into his office, he checked his records and asked me how my daughter was doing. I told him that she was fine, but that he had also delivered my son. He said, "But your son died!" Thank goodness it struck me funny. I responded that Robert seemed happy as he played with Jeannette when I left. The obstetrician felt bad, but he made my day! I believe he felt better about his mistake when he figured that out.

Taking long walks and singing lullabies to the babies was therapeutic for me. When weather allowed, the stroller rolled along many sidewalks in Richmond. I made some alterations on the stroller for Jeannette to accommodate the infant seat for Robert and off we went.

Although I sang in the church choir, performance was not my strong suit. I loved the fact that the babies calmed down when I sang to them. I sang all kinds of songs, but each child had a special lullaby. Robert's was "Acorn in the Meadow." I remember the words to this day.

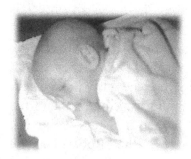

In the lullaby, a mother croons to her baby boy as she smiles down on him in his cradle. She compares his growth to an oak tree that begins as an acorn in the meadow. Her baby will become a "giant man" as the oak tree stretches to the sky.

Without a doubt, Robert grew to be a giant man—Perhaps not in stature, but in all the ways that truly matter in life.

Chapter 4

Sweetheart, I Am Not Asking You to Marry Me to Have Children

I've shared the beginning of Robert's part of the journey. Now I need to fill you in on my background as it contributes to this story.

My Background

The same year I was born my father graduated from Purdue University with a degree in Mechanical Engineering. Immediately after he graduated, he started working for American Blower Corporation. We moved frequently as he worked his way up in the company. We moved back and forth between Detroit, New York City, Toledo, and Columbus, Ohio. Then my parents, my younger sister, Jan, and I, moved back to Indianapolis when I was ten and a half.

Before we moved to Indianapolis permanently, we made frequent trips back to visit both sets of grandparents. I remember staying with my father's parents (Mom and Pop Esterline) in their very large home on North Meridian Street. My father and I would take morning walks up Meridian Street. I remember passing a mansion that had cement walls back from the sidewalk with a huge lawn between the walls and the mansion behind. My father explained that the man had built the wall to block the sounds from the street because his wife was mentally ill, and the noise bothered her. It was the first time I heard about mental illness.

A month or so after we moved back, my mother took Jan and me downtown to the Indianapolis Athletic Club (IAC) to swim. Jim Clark taught me to swim and started entering me in meets that same summer. I swam and dived for IAC and Coach Clark until I was nineteen years old.

Years later, I wrote an article that was published in the *Indianapolis Star Magazine* that read in part:

> *"In the '50's we could not swim for schools. Those of us who competed did so for private clubs, public pools, or community centers. Many Indianapolis kids in those days swam for Jim Clark and the Indianapolis Athletic Club...We called him King of the Coaches...*
>
> *"He gave each of us a chance to compete. Sometimes that meant risking a loss of points. He spent as much time (sometimes even more) with kids who had physical handicaps and would never turn a point as he did with his championship people...*
>
> *"He had many ways of letting each of us know our importance. When the team won by a point, he found one of us who had scored a single point. 'Yours was the one that won for us,' he'd say."*

Jim Clark was rare among coaches, especially at that time, because he was successful in coaching both men and women. He sent swimmers, both men and women, to the Olympic Games in 1952, 1956 and 1960. My experience as an athlete prepared me for life in more ways than I could ever imagine. To this day I am imbued with Coach Clark's emphasis on teamwork.

Although I liked being a girl, I was a tomboy. As I matured, I became more and more convinced that I would probably not marry. That fact concerned my parents because marriage was a social expectation at the time. A woman's success came through the success of her husband and sons. For me, loving a man and being tempted to marry was not a problem, but in the rationale of that day, a woman gave up her independence and lost everything, including her last name, when she married. Along with a growing conviction that I would not marry came a decision that I would not give birth to children of my own. I loved kids, but in that day single women who reared children were usually mothers who were widowed young. Then I met Ralph.

Meeting Ralph

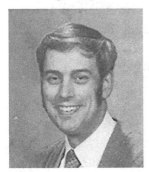

It was a Sunday evening in February 1960 at a singles' get-together at church. I had not been attending the singles' group although I had been active in the life of that church since I was a child. My grandfather was one of the founders, so we had great family involvement. The minister's wife invited me to join her for this occasion.

It was a dinner in which the guys were cooks for the girls. After dinner I saw that the cooks were also doing the cleanup—washing dishes and such. I told them that I would go down the hall to get my shoes which I had taken off and would be back in a few minutes to help.

I took off down the hall and found a man standing near the place where I had left my shoes. I recognized him, from the choir loft on Sunday mornings, as the same man who sat with Dr. Claude Otten and his wife Lois. Dr. Otten was a staff physician at the Methodist Hospital where I worked.

Ralph started a conversation, but I cut it a bit short, explaining that I had promised to help the men with the dishes. He said he would join me, and we went back together and started washing dishes. The minister's wife, who had attended a concurrent meeting, came to get me because she was going home. Ralph called me the next day to invite me for a date that Friday night. He told me there was a movie he wanted to see and a restaurant that his cousin recommended where we would eat. I accepted.

When Ralph drove up to the house, my little sister Mary and her friend Mary Ellen, who was spending the night, were watching out the front window. When Ralph eased himself out from behind the wheel of the VW Bug he was driving, they started giggling to see such a tall man get out of such a tiny car. When I opened the door to greet him, I said right away, "Ralph this is my sister Mary, and her friend Mary Ellen." Ralph replied, "I have a sister, Rosemary."

Next, we went to the kitchen and I introduced him to my mother. "Mother this is Ralph Lafuze; Ralph, this is my mother, Dorothy." Ralph replied, "My mother's name is Dorothy." Next, I said, "I can't introduce you to my sister Jan because she isn't home." Ralph replied, "I have a sister Jan."

We were driving around looking for the restaurant that his cousin recommended. She had not realized it was closed on Friday nights. It was a steakhouse owned and operated by a devout Catholic family that did not eat red meat on Fridays.

Ralph asked me how long I had worked at the Methodist Hospital. His uncle Claude, Dr. Otten, was on staff there, so it did not surprise me at all that he knew I worked there. I replied, "I can tell you exactly because I was hired on my birthday and started working three days later. So, it was August third."

There was a silence. "When is your birthday?" he asked. "July 31st," I said. Then there was a longer silence. "You are not going to believe this, but my birthday is July 31st." He was right. I questioned whether he was handing me a line, but it didn't matter. He was just a date. Only later when I came to know him well did I know that even though I did not always agree with him, I knew he was telling what he believed to be true. I never heard him tell a lie.

Ralph's Background

Ralph grew up on a farm north of Liberty, Indiana. His mother said that the only part of farming that Ralph liked was building fences. He loved structures like large dams and bridges. In his first year at Purdue he learned surveying, which he put to good use earning money for tuition and investing it as a student both at Purdue and IU. His degree was in Engineering Law that is no longer offered by Purdue. The engineering component was in Civil Engineering. The degree was contingent on taking three years of Civil Engineering at Purdue and three years of law school at Indiana University Bloomington. The degree was only granted at the end of Law School. So, in the spring of 1956 Ralph graduated from Purdue one weekend and IU Bloomington the next.

At that time there was a mandatory draft. He knew he'd be drafted when he graduated from law school. All his friends in the Navy urged him to join the Navy, and all his friends in the Army agreed. So, he joined the Navy. After Officer Candidate School he was assigned to Judge Advocate General (JAG) in Washington D.C. He was very happy there, and it was a good fit for him. One day the lieutenant in charge called him in and asked, "Ensign Lafuze, how would you like to go to Turkey?"

Ralph explained to me years later that he replied, "I wouldn't, Sir." According to Ralph's account, the lieutenant proceeded to convince him that all his life Ralph had dreamed of going to Turkey. The situation was that the base in Turkey was in the process of being built and there were limited bachelors' quarters with no provisions for accompanying wives and children.

Ralph was not married and uniquely qualified for that assignment. So, he served nineteen months as a legal officer on an Air Force Base in Karamürsel, Turkey. After that assignment, his reward was being able to choose from nearly unlimited possibilities. He chose an assignment as close to his Liberty, Indiana, home as possible. He served the remainder of his four-year military obligation at a Navy base in Crane, Indiana.

Over the years that Ralph practiced law, he was called upon to serve special judgeships. He enjoyed those assignments very much and his services were appreciated. The situations reminded me of his JAG appointment and where it could have led had he remained in the court system. Then I think again. If he had remained with JAG, we might never have met.

Ralph's Proposal

In March Ralph asked me to marry him and I heard myself saying, "Yes." In fact, what I sensed was that this was the person God wanted me to say yes to. I had not planned to marry or have children so my first words after saying yes were, "But you need to know that I plan not to have children." Ralph replied, "Sweetheart, I am not asking you to marry me to have children." We were married in October of 1960 and proceeded to have four babies in five years and three months. In fairness, birth control then was not as effective as birth control is now.

Chapter 5

The Pinmakers

L et me start my introduction to my grandfather, Pop, through the eyes of a reporter for The Indianapolis Star.

Introduction to Pop

This article appeared in the *Indianapolis Star* in April 1962:

> It was a cold, blustery day in March 1962. A radio announcement came in saying that the flight of Lt. Colonel John H. Glenn had been postponed again because of technical difficulties.
>
> Someone remarked that those missiles must be complicated structures. I knew they must be since in a local television broadcast the day before, the president of The Esterline Angus Instrument Company, located here in Indianapolis, had said that several hundred instruments made by his company were in use at Cape Canaveral. These instruments, he said, are used to record the functioning of the numerous automatic devices which control the missile.

I had a hunch that there might be the basis for a story within the walls of this sixty year old company. The next day, when I visited the plant and began to make inquiry, I discovered that there were a number of "firsts" in the history of this institution. This company operated the first plant in America for the commercial manufacture of permanent magnets. They developed the first six-volt electric starter for automobiles. During World War II, they made the instruments which enabled the United States Navy to clear the Atlantic Ocean of enemy submarines. I learned, too, that the founder of the company, John W. Esterline, had a remarkable football record at Purdue University, in spite of the fact that he is the lightest man ever to play a regular position on a major college football team.

When I began to probe into these early activities, it was clear that the men whom I was questioning were rather hazy about things that happened before they were born. I talked to Mr. Donald J. Angus, Mr. Esterline's associate for more than fifty years. When I asked him about the electric starter, he said that while the work on the starting system was going on, he was engaged in designing and building two electric light and power plants for Mr. Esterline, and that the man to see was Mr. Esterline himself. I called him on the telephone and asked whether I might see him to get some background for a story on the instruments being used at Cape Canaveral. He would see me at his home at any time that was convenient for me.

It was late afternoon when I drew up to a spacious Italian style home on North Meridian Street. I was here to meet the man who sixty years ago had founded the company I had visited the day before. At the door I was greeted by a man who will be eighty-eight next November. His weight will not exceed one hundred sixty pounds. He stood straight as an arrow. All of him is bone and muscle, no excess tissue. His hair is silvery gray. A high forehead rises from heavy brows which shelter a pair of deep-set hazel brown eyes. Like most men of a mechanical bent, he has an ample nose and a mouth that is firm. Despite his age, his face shows very few wrinkles. He gives me the impression of a man who has lived with a purpose.

He knew what I had come for, but seemingly tried to shift the conversation away from himself. When I told him about my children, he said, "Before you go, remind me to give you some notes on 'How to study.' It may help them in school." When I told him that my wife is interested in art, he replied, "That is fine. Encourage her," and he led me into the living room to see two large oil paintings of American Beech by Eyden. He said he had dabbled in art a little. When I expressed a desire to see some of his work, he said, "They are all wrapped up and in closets. You bring your wife out some evening, and we will get them out and talk about art."

Finally, I got around to the purpose of my visit. We talked for two hours. I found out how he happened to become interested in athletics, particularly football. How, after four years at Fort Wayne College (now Taylor University), he went to Purdue University because he was interested in engineering and football. How after graduation he was given a position as student instructor in order that he might play an additional year on the football team.

Later, while teaching at Purdue, he conceived the idea of the recording instrument and began its development. This was followed by the electric starter, "Golden Glow" fog penetrating headlights, permanent magnets, and the submarine device. I left with the impression that he considers the employees' profit-sharing plan which he and Mr. Angus developed, and which has been in effect for forty-five years, their crowning achievement.

He gave me permission to print my stories on his football career and the electric starter. Then I asked him why he had never written an autobiography.

"I've been too busy. I may try it when I get time," he replied.

April 1962   Fred B. Cavinder

The Pinmakers Meet

We drove down the long driveway to the mansion that my grandfather (all the family called him Pop) built for my grandmother (Mom to the family) for her 50th birthday. The red brick of the Mediterranean house and the red tile roof matched the small, red Volkswagen that Ralph drove. The house dwarfed our tiny car.

We parked in the drive and carried Robert up the steps leading to the front entrance. I loved coming home to Pop's house. The warmth of the red brick covered with ivy welcomed us. The terrace that ran the length of the house had once held all kinds of plants. I especially loved the lily-of-the-valley at the end of the terrace that Mom had planted and treasured years before.

We rang the bell and Dorothy, who had helped Pop and his only daughter, Margaret, for years answered. We hugged and exchanged greetings. Pop was in the library and hidden from our sight because the door was offset from the entrance. I loved the library and so did Pop. He sat under the lamp right around the corner from the door.

The comfortable leather chair showed its age more than Pop his. Margaret sat in the opposite corner listening to her radio and gazing out the window. Among Pop's many endeavors was the nursery he owned that was now run by his oldest son and family. The numerous plants and trees of all varieties on the property added to the landscape. I remember having the most impressive leaf collections several years in school. Each had as its nucleus leaves from Pop's trees. The one I remember most was the pink dogwood that peeked around the corner of the library window. The dark wood paneling may have seemed oppressive to some, but to me it was like a womb that held me as a child in a safe, warm place to explore books and magazines that took me around the world. It was to this almost sacred place that Ralph and I brought our son.

When we came into the library, Pop looked up from whatever he was reading and smiled. Pop was an amazing person. I never tired of his stories—even at their repeated telling. He talked about growing up the oldest of six boys. He remembered telling his mother there were too many babies and how bad he felt when she responded, "Walter, I don't know which one I would send back." She had a daughter, also. Her last pregnancy resulted in twins—a boy and a girl. Pop quoted her, "I finally got my girl, but I had to take another boy with her."

Pop's second-grade teacher told him not to quit school—keep going as far as you can she told him. He stayed through high school and finally made it to Purdue University. He was small and scrappy. He stood 5 feet 3 inches or so and weighed a little more than 140 pounds soaking wet, but he loved athletics. He played football for Purdue. As a quarterback he perfected a drop kick (which is illegal now). It was a surprise tactic because he could recover the ball farther down the field after he kicked it.

In 1897 he graduated from Purdue University in a brand-new discipline called electrical engineering. He taught engineering and was athletic director at Purdue for several years. He left Purdue to start his own company in Lafayette, Indiana, but it did not survive the floods of 1914.

The generosity of pioneers at the Indianapolis Motor Speedway brought him to Indianapolis. Carl Fisher and James Allison provided a building in Speedway that he could use and the Esterline company was born. In later years he formed a partnership with D. J. Angus, and the name of the company changed to Esterline Angus.

When Pop died fifteen years after he retired, there were people who had worked at Esterline Angus who came to pay their respects. I remember well one elderly gentleman who said, "During the depression when everyone was poor, at times Mr. Esterline didn't take pay, but there was always something in each of our pay envelopes."

Why am I telling you about our visit with Pop that day? Pop told me the story I had heard many times; about how small he was when he was born. "The chicken scale said I was two pounds and something. They did not think I would live, but I did. I remember as a boy hearing a neighbor ask my dad, 'Bill, what are you going to do with that runt?' My father answered, 'Walter will be our pinmaker.'" I knew the story well, but this time Pop added a line, "Don't you worry about this one. Robert will be your pinmaker."

When I have mentioned the pinmaker story to others over the years, the obvious question I get in response is, "What in the world is a pinmaker?" I answer that I have no idea what a pinmaker is. The only two I have known who were given that name were my son and grandfather. Both started life as tiny babies who were not expected to live. In adulthood, they both remained small in stature and build. Neither tried to draw attention to himself. In fact, they were just the opposite. The two pinmakers I have known were "giant men" in small bodies whose lives have made a difference in the world.

Pop did start that book which he titled, "The Pinmaker."
He was unable to finish it, but my sister Mary McGarvey did a
beautiful job of typing chapters from his notes and assembling
the remainder of his projected format. Her efforts to publish
The Pinmaker have not been successful thus far, but we will
continue those efforts.

Chapter 6

The First Ear Specialist

A s Robert grew, he continued having ear problems. When he was eighteen months old, the pediatrician referred us to an ear, nose, and throat specialist in Richmond. The pediatrician explained to me that Robert had fluid behind his ear drum that was taking too long to be absorbed between ear infections. "He is too young and too small right now for the surgery to insert tubes, but that may be the ultimate solution. I want for you to establish a relationship with the specialist so he can keep an eye on the situation as Robert progresses."

I was surprised when the specialist examined Robert's ears and claimed, "Mother, we can help this child. We'll schedule surgery to insert tubes as soon as possible." Then he showed me a message he planned to send to the pediatrician indicating that Robert had what is now called "Intellectual Disability."

I did not say a word to the specialist but questioned the pediatrician as to how the specialist had determined that. The pediatrician assured me that he had not said anything in the referral to indicate such a finding. He suggested that often when an eighteen-month-old's weight was as low as Robert's there were intelligence delays.

So, Robert had ear surgery on February 4, 1965. I remember the day vividly because it was the day the Richmond phone company burned, and the city was left without phone service.

Police had to patrol the streets checking specially designated homes to see if residents needed assistance because they could not phone for help.

Robert's surgery went well despite the lack of phone service. The success of the surgery was evident on the drive home when Robert needed the radio volume turned down. His childish "tattoo" changed to "thank you." One of the doctors where I worked Saturdays to help pay for Robert's care commented on his bright eyes. Robert was normally intelligent. He tested in the normal range in kindergarten.

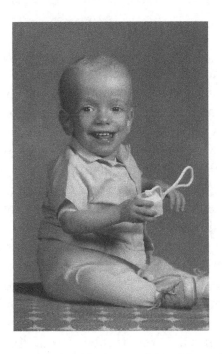

At 18 months, Robert grinned broadly
and we all smiled back.

Chapter 7

The Power of Stigma

All our family, including her grandchildren, called my grandmother Esterline "Mom." She died when I was nine years old. I remember her well. She was a high-school graduate, which was quite an accomplishment for girls in her day.

When she was diagnosed with cancer, it was considered a dirty, filthy disease that people did not talk about. When a famous person such as a movie star or politician died of cancer, it was mentioned in the obituary as an unconfirmed, unknown, or undiagnosed illness.

Part of the reason it was "hush hush" was because there was no known cause. Worse yet, the public was unaware of any scientific explanation. This created an atmosphere of fear. It was sometimes seen as a curse, a punishment for sin, much like leprosy in biblical times.

When Mom had a recurrence, I was six years old and devastated. I remember praying that she would live. She did not want my grandfather to tell the second doctor about her earlier experience with cancer. Pop retired to take care of her the rest of her life.

What I have explained is my first understanding of the negative power of stigma. How ironic that as a young adult I lived to see the progress we have made as the power of stigmatized cancer was conquered. This happened through scientific discoveries made after prominent people announced to the public that they had cancer. Some established foundations to educate the public and find cures. I consider those people heroes.

Even more ironic is the fact that I had a son who was finally diagnosed with an illness that is even more stigmatizing than cancer. My former research collaborator in pediatric hematology/oncology, Dr. Jeffrey Goldman, died of brain cancer. His memorial service was at Riley Hospital where we had our research lab, and where he treated cancer patients until several weeks before he died. His memorial service program had a verse about all those things that cancer cannot take away. Schizophrenia lacks that kind of mercy. It takes everything and teaches the lessons of loss. We have learned them well. Robert learned them even better.

Through my experience with Robert I met my friend and colleague, Bernice Pescosolido, an Indiana University Bloomington professor of Sociology who received her Ph.D. from Yale University and has dedicated her career to studying and researching stigma. Among her other accomplishments, Dr. Pescosolido established an interdisciplinary consortium for research related to mental illnesses that included Indiana University faculty but reached far beyond to other universities and other states.

Organizations such as The National Alliance on Mental Illness (NAMI) and Mental Health America (MHA) have brought us a long way in reducing the stigma associated with mental illnesses such as schizophrenia, bipolar illness, and depression, but we are not "there" yet. The stigma associated with mental illness paralyzes progress.

Chapter 8

We Are Not Here to Assign Blame. We Are Here to Solve Problems.

Meanwhile, our family was increasing in size. Having four babies in five years and three months was a challenge, but somehow it was easier rearing them than if I had planned it. I think that is because I had no pre-conceived ideas of what I wanted for them. Ralph and I loved each one in the same way, and we loved each one in a unique way. We met needs and solved problems as they arose.

I learned early that if I needed to talk on the phone or concentrate on a problem, it was more effective to call a name and ask that person to move to another place than give a general request to all of the kids to quiet down. At first the one whose name I had called would say, "Mom, it wasn't my fault." I

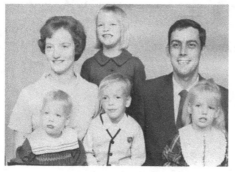

would respond, "We are not here to assign blame, we are here to solve problems." I was careful to call on a different child each time making the rounds. Once they caught on, they trusted that there was truly no effort on my part to assign blame. The calling of a name with the request to move please became a signal that I needed quiet for some task that I was performing.

I have lived long enough to reap the reward of those early efforts. For example, when our youngest daughter Mary was on summer vacation one year, I gave her clear instructions that when she visited Robert who was at Larue Carter Hospital, she could do me a favor. She herself, as an outpatient, had an appointment with a Larue Carter psychiatrist. She had a block of time between inpatient visiting hours and her appointment.

As a favor to me she was to pick up a survey I had written and left with the receptionist at Larue Carter Hospital. Later she told me that she could not do the favor because the receptionist did not have the survey. I dismissed it, thinking for some reason she did not want to do it. I was wrong.

The next time she and I had a conversation Mary told me, "I'm sorry, Mom, but the receptionist at Riley Hospital did not have the survey." I responded that I was sure I had told her the receptionist at Larue Carter. She explained further, "Yes, but in your follow-up email, you said Riley Hospital." I checked my email, and sure enough in my message to her I had written Riley. I apologized and told her it was my fault. In a matter-of-fact voice I heard my daughter respond, "Mom, we are not here to assign blame, we are here to solve problems." Yes, I thought. They do listen and learn from us.

The second method I developed of working with the kids as a team was by developing The Captain System. This scheme had its rules. First, I need to explain that we did not have an inclined plane when our kids stood side by side. Jeannette was taller than the other three, who were about the same height. Besides, the oldest daughter was very well organized and could have run the household by the time she was six.

I was entrenched in the team concept by my coach, Jim Clark. Jim would say, "We swim as a team or we don't swim." I did not want Jeannette to become the "Bossy Big Sister." So here comes the Captain System.

The captain rotated each week. It was up to the kids to keep track of who was captain. They kept a calendar that Jeannette remembers to this day. I used the system when I was in class or otherwise unable to be with the kids. The captain did not participate in the activities. The captain oversaw knowing where each member of the team was and keeping them together. If there was spending money involved, the captain held onto the money and made sure each person got a fair share. When we began, the youngest was barely four. As I told Ralph, I knew why I devised the system. First, they realized from the beginning that they were in this together and that cooperating with the captain would result in returned cooperation. Even more, when I had a need for heavy responsibility and asked, "Where is my captain," the smallest hand went up.

To this day, our kids work together as a team. I praise God as the inspiration for the Captain System. Coach Clark, wherever you are, you get credit, too.

Chapter 9

Robert Goes to School

I noticed that Robert often substituted one word for another. It seemed like such a small issue at the time but looking back, I wonder whether it might have been an early clue that his brain might be different. The example that I noticed most when I visited pre-school was that Robert answered roll call by saying "president," rather than, "present."

Pre-School

Robert attended a pre-school where he thrived in some ways but had difficulty in others. His pre-school teacher advised us to wait an extra year to send him to kindergarten. I asked my friend, who was a kindergarten teacher at the time, whether we would have legal problems when Robert was six years old and not in the first grade. She assured us that the system would recognize the fact that he was in a continuing-education system, but just a year behind.

At the time we had no idea how positive the results of that decision would be. Robert was fully eighteen when he had his break with reality, but we were spared by the fact that he had not left home for college. In sharing with friends whose sons have had breaks from reality after they left home, we realize how blessed we were to have been spared that hurdle.

Kindergarten

Robert went to afternoon kindergarten just as his older sister had. He was ready in most ways, but he was resistant to any change. In our district, kindergarten was a half day. We carpooled with several neighbors to take the children to school, and the bus brought them home. One neighborhood mom shared with me that Robert did not want to go in when there had been a substitute teacher the day before. She had to walk in with him. As luck would have it that mom was the only one of the three of us who had that happen. I had been totally unaware. However, as I thought about it, Robert did resist change.

The second challenge we had was that either I needed to meet him at the bus when the driver stopped to let him off, or the driver had to help him down the bus steps. The next year when Robert rode the bus both ways, the driver helped him on and off the bus. As the driver put it, "It simply isn't cool from a young man's perspective to have his mom help him on and off the school bus."

One of the kindergarten teacher's remarks sticks in my mind to this day. When meeting with me about Robert's progress she said, "To determine his true IQ I would have to administer a separate IQ test that would take half a day at least. There is no way that I can do that here. All I can give you are these test results, which place him well above normal."

I did not realize how important his IQ level would be as he passed through the system and beyond. It was not because we really cared about his IQ, (we have no idea what our daughters' IQs are). It is because the mental-illness system equates IQ with developmental disorders generally. Intellectual Deficiency is a part of the evaluation classification. In a perfect world we would distinguish between the two. It is not because we demand a perfect world but providing services for someone who has a normal or above IQ, however badly compromised by illness or medications, has different possible outcomes.

First and Second Grades

Robert had the same teacher for first and second grade. She was able to do very well with him. The comment I remember most was, "Robert is an excellent reader." One of his saddest losses after his break with reality came when he was prescribed strong doses of anticholinergic medications. Those kinds of medications impaired his ability to focus his eyes, and his ability to read was severely impaired. When medical complications forced doctors to discontinue his anticholinergic medication Robert was profoundly psychotic, but he could read perfectly. I heard him read from a photo tribute to his father who had died several years earlier. It was a verse from Romeo and Juliet. He read every word, including William Shakespeare, perfectly. What a trade-off to have to juggle between psychosis and the ability to read.

I also noticed that Robert did not respond to cues well. At some point he started asking people, "Are you mad at me?" Although this question began in childhood, it persisted throughout his adult life. Some people were perplexed by his questioning, others were hurt, and some offended. I finally figured out that because he could not read the cues from peoples' faces or body language that many of us can, he was uncertain about when to stop talking or change the subject. The last thing that he wanted was for someone to become angry with him.

Third Grade

When Robert was in third grade, he had a teacher whom we barely knew at the beginning of the year. She and her husband had recently moved their membership from another town to our church. Over that year we became good friends through church activities.

Very close to the beginning of the third grade, Robert's teacher took the class on a school bus from Hagerstown to downtown Indianapolis. At that time the teacher barely knew us as a family. One of the adventures of the day was climbing to the top of the Monument Circle, which at that time may have been the tallest building in downtown Indianapolis. The teacher told us later that when they were close to the top, she heard one of Robert's classmates say that he hadn't kept up

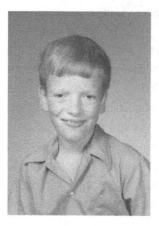

with the group and was still climbing. When Robert appeared, he was out of breath and could barely say, "Wait until I tell my dad." The teacher told us that she was concerned because she knew his dad was an attorney. Her concerns were relieved when she heard his next comment, "He will be so proud of me!"

During that year Robert had two breakthroughs at school. He was placed in her level for homeroom which was not the highest level. He was placed higher for math but there was a realization on the homeroom teacher's part that Robert had a hard time getting things ready to change rooms. For one thing he had to take a different book with him. For another he resisted changing rooms. She volunteered and we agreed to have him stay in her room for math.

The second thing we realized was that Robert couldn't hear. His teacher talked to me about it. "Joan, do you realize that Robert doesn't hear?" I countered that he had just had his hearing tested and it was normal. How could that be? His teacher replied, "Well you stand directly behind him and say something that requires his attention." I did as she suggested and got no response.

When I questioned the family-practice physician we had at the time, he explained that Robert was eager to succeed. The school audiologist must have inadvertently sent some message that Robert picked up. Either she set up a pattern that he could decipher or somehow changed her tone or made a movement that tipped him off. He raised his hand not by what he heard but rather by what he observed or sensed.

We had his hearing tested and he had a loss significant enough to warrant having a consult with an ear specialist. The specialist in Muncie examined him and reported holes in his eardrum due to neglect of repeated ear infections. The receptionist did not schedule a return appointment because the doctor was going to be out of his office for several months. Discouraged, I consulted with the family-practice physician who examined Robert's ears again. He assured me that the holes the specialist had seen were due to weak spots on his eardrum. They were left by previous insertion of tubes and had opened after his last examination of Robert's ears. He knew there was no neglect involved. All Robert had to do was touch his ear or complain of an ache and we were in his office. The specialist in Richmond was no longer in practice, so we were stumped.

Chapter 10

Dr. David E. Brown

Ralph's uncle, Claude, got us an appointment with Dr. David E. Brown whose office was just north of the Methodist Hospital in Indianapolis. Dr. Brown and Robert hit it off right away. Robert would go into his appointment and before he sat down, he would take everything out of his pockets and put the articles on a table beside him. Why? Either I did not know or do not remember. But I have no trouble remembering the action and even more I remember the patient smile on Dr. Brown's face.

He examined Robert's ears and ordered a hearing test. Then came the news. "I believe I can restore Robert's hearing in his left ear to normal. I will operate on the right ear because although I cannot restore it to normal, I want to restore it enough so that he will be able to track sound. That will be important to him." So, Robert was admitted to the old St. Vincent Hospital on Fall Creek Boulevard several times. It was a remarkable place. I had done most of my med-tech internship there, and it was like family.

The sacred sisters were in charge then and made places for employees. Everyone from the physicians and nurses right on up to the maintenance and housekeeping workers knew Robert by name and welcomed him when he came in for surgeries. In those days the surgeries involved elaborate packing, which was removed after six weeks. The first bandaging to hold it in place was immense and doubled Robert's head size. Before he went home, the outside packaging was reduced in size, but the internal packing was left for six weeks. One of the things that always amazed me was that Dr. Brown, who was obviously near-sighted, had a difficult time locating me in the waiting room. I smiled that the person who had such a struggle finding me in the waiting room had done such intricate surgery on my son.

The first surgery after Dr. Brown removed the packing and ordered the hearing test, he shook his head in disbelief at the results. He had Robert's hearing retested with a different audiologist. "I cannot believe it," he said. Not only was Robert's hearing normal in his left ear, but also his hearing in the right ear was above the normal line. Robert heard normally from then on.

The last surgery by Dr. Brown was after St. Vincent moved to its 86th Street location. By that time Robert had become quite a swimmer. He felt a freedom in the water that he loved. Even more, he loved being under water. After Dr. Brown found me in the waiting room that time, he told me that Robert's last words before he went under the anesthetic were, "Dr. Brown when can I swim again?" I believe I saw tears in Dr. Brown's eyes when he shook his head and whispered, "He will not be able to get water in his ears again. I'm so sorry."

When Robert came out of recovery I was shocked at the size of the external packaging. The bandaged package was even larger than before. Later when Doctor Brown was ready to go home at the end of the day, he stopped by to check on Robert once more. He was dressed in his street clothes and obviously on his way out. He looked at Robert and compassion filled his face.

"Robert, would you feel better if I made the bandage smaller?" Robert nodded yes. For him to change the bandaging that meant that Dr. Brown had to take off his jacket, page an assistant to bring sterile supplies, help him put on a sterile gown and gloves, and create a sterile field where he could remove the extra bandaging. When Dr. Brown finished the bandage was smaller and much more comfortable.

Not long after that, Dr. Brown moved to California to be close to family. It was several years later that Mother Lafuze brought a friend by who sat in our living room and shared information we did not know about Dr. David E. Brown. "I understand your son was a patient of Dr. David E. Brown." I nodded. "He was my husband's doctor until my husband died. Did you know that he had been Chair of the Ear Nose and Throat division of the IU School of Medicine until he retired to that private practice north of the Methodist Hospital?" I indicated I had not known that.

"You knew that he was in a terrible car accident at 46th and Washington Boulevard, didn't you?" I indicated I had not known that. "Well, a passerby pulled him out of the burning car and stayed with him until help came and disappeared into the crowd that had formed. Dr. Brown was burned so badly that they had to remove a kidney, but he recovered and continued to practice." I remember thinking that this kind, compassionate person who was so loving and patient with Robert must have known pain and suffering himself.

As have several others who treated Robert after his break with reality, Dr. David E. Brown did more than practice medicine. He and those others have practiced the kind of magic that heals beyond what practicing medicine can touch. Wherever they are today, accept the loving gratitude of Robert Lafuze's mother, Joan. Amen.

Chapter 11

Robert Continues His Journey Through School

Meanwhile, back at school Robert had entered the fourth grade. He had started to give alternative names to teachers with whom he had contact. Two names I remembered well were Mrs. Rice and Mr. Miller. Mr. Miller was a sixth-grade teacher who had the thankless and difficult job of keeping order in the school cafeteria. He did an excellent job. Robert was afraid of him. I am more than certain that Robert's perfect discipline in the cafeteria was fear-based. All these years later, I remember that Robert's name for Mr. Miller was Mr. Killer.

His name for his fourth-grade home room and social studies teacher Mrs. Rice was Mrs. Nice. He loved her. She was able to enhance his strengths and diminish his weaknesses. She sponsored a talent show and found a role for every member of her class. She appointed Robert the role of Master of Ceremonies. Robert was a natural extrovert, had a pleasant speaking voice and was a good reader. These were a perfect combination for the talent show Master of Ceremonies.

I also remember Robert's situation in math. His basic math skills were excellent. He did well with addition, subtraction, and multiplication—if you were willing to overlook timed tests. His success on those was variable, but he managed to pass them. His Bugga Bear was long division. However, he had been assured by his math teacher that he would be okay. Robert repeatedly said, "I am not good at long division, but he says not to worry. My teacher says not to worry that I can't do long division yet." I heard these kinds of statements almost every day until the fatal day that Robert came home and blurted out, "Mom, it's time to worry!"

I remember the day toward the end of the year when I went to school to talk with Mrs. Rice. I was concerned because even in the fourth grade Robert had a difficult time keeping up with all the teachers he had. He had a separate teacher for Math and Physical Education and Speech Therapy besides his home-room teacher. The way the school was structured he faced having nine separate teachers in the fifth grade.

When I entered the room and told Mrs. Rice I was concerned, she took over the conversation. "I am concerned about Robert next year, also. I am moving up a grade so he will be assigned to my homeroom, but he really needs a self-contained classroom. The only one we have now is for students who are intellectually challenged and that is not Robert's challenge. He has some intellectual advantages beyond his current placement. He pays a price for that. I wonder whether you could find a school system nearby that could meet Robert's needs."

Upper Elementary School: Hagerstown

When we talked with Robert about it, he was adamant. Of course, he did not want to change! He was happy where he was. So, we held our breath and prayed. Robert managed in the fifth grade. It was a challenge keeping up in the ways we anticipated, though.

Having Mrs. Rice as his home-room teacher helped; but then she became ill. She missed several days with pneumonia. After she returned to the classroom, Robert came home one day and reported that Mrs. Nice had shaken him by the shoulders. "It didn't hurt at all, Mom, but I don't know what I did to make her mad at me." I handled the situation by pinning a note to the back of Robert's shirt, "Robert told me that you were upset with something he did today, but he couldn't tell what he had done. Please let me know how to explain to Robert so he can correct whatever he did. He wasn't angry at all. He was just confused. We want to support you in every way."

That day a note came back from Mrs. Rice. "Mrs. Lafuze, Robert did nothing to deserve my response. I have been battling this pneumonia and I am not myself. I have told Robert I am sorry. It was my fault, but you please assure him also." Mrs. Rice did not have recurring pneumonia. She had lung cancer although she was a non-smoker. She was a person of faith. I heard a story that she had a vision that she would be healed. The story that I heard was that she was given an exact date in the vision, and her thought was that her healing miracle would be a celebration tribute to the power of God. In a strange way her vision came true. The reported date she was given was the day she died. Robert and I attended her celebration of life.

Sixth Grade in Richmond: Joseph Moore

Robert came home the last day of fifth grade and asked, "Remember Mom when you told me that I could go to another school last year? I am ready to try another school for the sixth grade." I realized his dilemma. He didn't want to leave Hagerstown, but he realized the challenge of the teachers he would have and the confusion of changing classes so often. We looked in New Castle and in Richmond. The superintendent of public schools in Richmond was more positive about meeting our needs and picked several possible schools and teachers to interview. Robert was the one who led the interviews. He picked Mr. Tim Williamson at Joseph Moore School. Mr. Williamson had similar skills to Mrs. Rice. He was able to enhance Robert's strengths and diminish his weaknesses.

I have three vivid memories of Robert's sixth-grade experience at Joseph Moore. The first day he came home and said that I needed to teach him how to tie shoes. When I talked to

Mr. Williamson, he explained that they had shoe-tying races in gym and Robert had trouble tying shoes. He still had a difficult time, so we ended up putting no-tie shoes on him for gym. He was already wearing loafers that did not require tying for everyday wear. The problem was the school would not allow street shoes on the gym floor.

The second event that Robert talked about often was the train trip they took as a class to Chicago. Robert had a great time. He already knew Chicago well because Ralph's sister, her husband, and daughter lived in a Chicago suburb at the time. Robert talked about that trip often over the years.

A third memory from sixth grade was a writing contest, "What Freedom Means to Me," which was sponsored by Seratoma, a service organization that was active in Richmond at that time. Mr. Williamson saw that contest as an opportunity for Robert and made sure that he guided Robert to success. The only reason I knew what Robert wrote was because the submission had to be in Robert's own handwriting.

Mr. Williamson talked to me about the submission, explaining what I already knew. Robert's handwriting left a lot to be desired. What he said was for me to sit with Robert and let him write one or two sentences at a time. It was slow-going, but it worked. Robert won the Joseph Moore contest.

The leaders in Seratoma talked with Mr. Williamson about Robert's entry. Mr. Williamson shared with me later that they had wanted to award Robert first place, but they wanted him to replace a phrase that he had used. He had referred at some point to "The Gates of Hell!" Mr. Williamson explained that if he had used the expression as a profanity that would have been different, but he had used it very appropriately and he refused to have Robert change it. So, Robert ended up with a second place. He received $5 for winning the Joseph Moore contest. That made him very happy.

What I remember from the essay all these years later was that Robert wrote about the positives of being free. I am sure that was where the Gates of Hell came in. It was probably a reference to the high price some pay so that we can enjoy being free to do almost anything we want. However, it was the other side of freedom that my son captured in a metaphor so graphic it makes me shiver to this day.

I must explain that Robert had heard Ralph's Aunt Lois talk about her granddaughter's friend who had gone to a slumber party. In those days the plate glass in patio doors broke into glass shards rather than crumbling as it is required to do now. One of the girls had gone through a plate glass patio door and severed her femoral artery. She bled to death before they could get it stopped. Robert asked question after question about severed arteries and how they could cause death.

I remember the line in his Seratoma Essay that read: "Freedom can be like a severed artery." Who is this man-child I call my son, I asked myself?

Back to Hagerstown for 7ᵗʰ Grade

We were advised that no junior high school in Richmond would be more appropriate, so he went to the seventh grade in Hagerstown. Robert managed, but there were no arrangements for his learning differences. For example, handwriting has always been a challenge for Robert and for Ralph and me. I am not certain about the reason for Ralph, but even his secretaries had trouble deciphering his scribble.

Robert's was probably due to his muscle weakness and possibly other issues. I know why mine was at least unorthodox. I missed cursive-writing instruction which was taught in the third grade in my school, because I had many common childhood diseases. Today there are vaccines that prevent those diseases. I not only had those diseases in the third grade, but I had barely recovered from the flu when I came down with scarlet fever. My handwriting is a unique blend of cursive-print.

When Robert was in the seventh grade, he had a teacher who was very strict about handwriting. By that time, we had Robert using a keyboard. He was typing assignments successfully. This teacher insisted that he turn in handwritten work. When we met the teacher at parent/teacher meetings, we brought up the subject for discussion. The teacher explained his position on the importance of using handwriting. He said that Robert had given him the explanation for his challenges by saying that bad handwriting runs in my family. He made this statement although all three of his sisters have very acceptable handwriting. I responded by saying that Robert should not have made such a smart-aleck remark. The teacher replied seriously and with a very straight face. "Oh, it was not a smart-aleck response. Robert was very serious." Ouch!

Always a Friend

When Robert needed a friend, he had a friend. In fact, he had a way of making friends. I noticed that Robert protected himself coming home from grade school. Out our back window I could watch Robert and his friends start across the football field behind our house on the other side of the creek. Then as they came to the footbridge over the creek, he found something interesting in the grass and leaned over to pick up a stone or some other small object.

The reason he stopped was because the footbridge had no handrails on either side. It was a favorite pastime for the boys to wrestle on the bridge to see who could stay on the bridge and who ended up in the water. Robert protected himself from that kind of horseplay. He knew what the outcome would be. Robert waited until the boys had started up the hill that led to our property before he hurried across the bridge to join them.

But there was one boy who lived next door to us who was the biggest and brawniest of all. I believe he became a fire-fighter. His name is most appropriate, Rocky. Robert trusted Rocky to keep him safe and walked across the footbridge with Rocky when he was there.

One Friday Rocky spent the night at our house. The next morning the two boys decided to walk down the back forty, across the footbridge and the football field either to play on the playground or to walk on into town. I watched from the kitchen window as they left down the back forty. Robert stopped as they got a short distance from the footbridge. I wondered what had happened. Had Robert lost his trust in Rocky?

I could see them talking. Robert turned around and started up the slope to home, but Rocky called something to him. What in the world is happening, I wondered? My concerns were quelled when, in the next few moments, I saw Rocky take off his sweater and help Robert put it on. Robert had realized that he was cold and needed a jacket. Thank you, God for sending angels like Rocky.

Chapter 12

Burris

Through testing we were able to discover that Robert had a learning disability that affected processing what he heard. This learning disability is like dyslexia for some persons who have reading differences. It told us he could learn, but it was a different way of learning. When he was ready for the eighth grade, we tried to find a school that would meet his special learning needs.

The answer was Muncie Burris, a statewide school associated with Ball State University in Muncie. There was no tuition, but we had to provide transportation. It was a 30-mile trip that took a minimum of forty-five minutes to get to Burris, which was on the far side of Muncie from Hagerstown. Getting him to school and back was a true challenge. At the time I was no longer attending school at Ball State in Muncie. I had been accepted to the doctoral program in physiology at the Indiana University School of Medicine in Indianapolis.

Many days I would drive Robert to Muncie to Burris School and wait for the building to open at 6:30 a.m. Then I headed to Indianapolis to meet my graduate-school responsibilities. Later in the day, I reversed the circuit to pick Robert up at Burris and return home to Hagerstown. The round-trip meant four-and-a-half to five hours on the road. Now and then we had help. A teacher for one of the Muncie schools from Hagerstown went out of his way to pick Robert up and take him to school as often as he could. We also had a friend who went to Muncie for classes at Ball State who would occasionally bring him home.

When Robert turned sixteen, he began to drive himself. I believe that was his last year at Burris, but it was a huge relief. Sometimes when the weather was too bad for him to drive, one of us would take him, but Robert did well with driving; even though our cars were stick-shift, he could do it.

The set-up at Burris was that all students were main-streamed. However, there was a special classroom to meet the needs of students with learning differences. Robert used that classroom for typing and later for math. He did well with basic math skills but had trouble with abstract math. That led to serious problems with algebra. The solution was to add math in the resource room to his schedule.

Another experience I remember from Burris was meeting with his eighth-grade science teacher. She was great. She was young, relatively new at teaching and brought the energy of youth into the classroom. She liked Robert and he liked her.

Her first words to me were, "Your son is a cop-out." I didn't have to wait long to know what she meant. She explained quickly. "Look at these two tests. On the first one Robert missed all but a few of the questions. All he had to do for this one was look at the board and write down the answers on the paper."

Well, that did not surprise me at all. Robert's muscles never developed appropriately. I explained to her that passing that test required overcoming most challenges Robert had. It required him to look away from his paper, refocus his eye muscles to the board to read the words, refocus his eyes on the paper and write the answer there with muscles in his fingers that made handwriting difficult. A few iterations of that cycle would bring two F words to mind: Fatigue and Failure. Exclude Focus and Fun.

Then she proceeded to show me his physics test over the subject of light. "Robert had no problem with this one. He got the second highest grade in the class. On this one he had to follow the lecture and figure out the answers for himself. It was not one that I gave answers to. Look at how well he did. He only missed one of them."

I could not explain that to her, but trust me, I did not rush out to tell Robert he was a cop-out. Instead I told him that at my parent/teacher conference with his science teacher she had told me he had done well on his physics test on light. His response made me smile. "Oh, Mom, that was easy. Grandpa Esterline explained all that when he gave me his camera." I could picture the scene. My mind saw my father, the mechanical engineer, sitting with his beloved grandson explaining the camera that he was now giving him because Robert was fascinated with it. All these years later, I can picture my father as he pointed to the different parts of the camera. Perhaps he even paused for a moment and found a way to draw a picture or two as he continued his explanation. God, thank you for giving Robert a loving supportive family so that he could teach us how to achieve true joy in living!

Robert made friendships at Burris that lasted after he came back to Hagerstown. One afternoon when Robert was at Burris, I came to pick him up, but I had to go into the building to drop something off. As I walked down the hall, I heard voices from the top of the stairwell, "Hey Robert! Are you headed back to Beggarstown?"

It was friendly banter. I heard Robert reply in the positive as I climbed the steps part way. There I saw Robert standing above two boys on the stairs below him. They were obviously friends sharing a happy after-school moment. Later, I met their family who took Robert in to provide a "home away from home" for him. The boys' mother made an autumn wreath that I have kept, remembering that family and their kindness to Robert. As I recall that first meeting, I noticed how carefully Robert protected himself by standing above them on the stairway. He was always careful to protect his vulnerability.

Chapter 13

Robert Taught Us the Most Important Lessons in Life

I look at pictures of Robert when he was in pre-school and marvel at how happy he was. He was the only one of the six of us who was clearly extroverted. He seemed to gain energy from being around other people. When other people weren't around, he seemed to gain energy from the world around him and being alive.

Which is Farther? Heaven or Florida?

His questions came one after another. One of his childhood questions was the inspiration for the title of this book. "Mom, I know that Dad gave me my name, Robert, but Mom, what I really want to ask is how Dad knew that was the name God wanted for me?" Many of his questions I have forgotten because they were straight-forward and easy to answer, but others left me stumped. "Mom, which is bigger, a palace or a mansion?" I tried by answering that there were smaller and larger of each.

One early evening, Robert pulled me outside to see what he described as looking like a big fish. It was a dead rabbit that I explained may have been caught by a dog and run over by a car. That prompted a question in response that made me smile, remembering how many professors had answered questions with new questions. "Mom, which runs faster, a rabbit or a dog?"

Once Robert asked, "Mom, how come you say, 'I don't know' so much?" The question he had asked to get that response was, "Mom, which is farther, Heaven or Florida?" Ralph told me that I might as well have said Heaven because he had a better chance of getting there. I must explain that Robert was young enough at the time that Ralph was struggling to establish an infant law practice. Years later, Robert's youngest sister, Mary, wrote a poem to answer the question. (A copy of the poem, just as she wrote it, is at the back of this book.) She claimed he was such a good person that he was much closer to Heaven than Florida. For many reasons her small "Big Brother" was her hero.

We Were Robert's Guests at a Hagerstown vs Burris Basketball Game

Three other memories of Mary's fierce loyalty to Robert stand out. When he was in high school at Muncie Burris it happened that the Hagerstown Boys Basketball team played a game at Burris. Robert invited us as his guests. Our family sat with him in the Burris fans' cheering section. Mary said with pride, "If anyone asks me why I was sitting with Burris fans, I will tell them that my big brother is a Burris student, and we were his guests."

Mary Becomes a NAMI "Consumer"

It was almost a decade later when Mary was officially diagnosed with Panic Disorder. She had her first episode when she was a junior in high school. Both she and I were concerned that she was experiencing the beginning stages of Robert's illness. I was on the phone immediately with Robert's psychiatrist at the time. After hearing my description of Mary's episode, he assured me that I could make an appointment with him at any time, but he felt her situation was different from Robert's. It was several years later when her symptoms became severe enough to warrant a visit to the psychiatrist for treatment.

Mary was grateful to Robert for leading our way into understanding the biological basis of both of their mental illnesses. She was grateful for our affiliation with what is now The National Alliance on Mental Illness (NAMI) for its emphasis on support, education, advocacy, and the importance of brain-based research. She readily identified as a "consumer," which is NAMI's term for a person who has a diagnosis of one of the brain-based illnesses our culture calls mental illnesses. I have told both of my children who have psychiatric diagnoses that I would abide by their wishes on remaining silent about their illnesses. Both have given me permission to talk freely. Robert said over and over, "Mom if someone can learn about what this is like, you talk and talk and talk!"

Mary and Robert made a great teaching team. Robert was treated with both medication and Electroconvulsive Therapy (ECT) for schizophrenia and mood disorder. Often, I mentioned to a psychiatrist that I thought he also had panic and anxiety as well as being on the autism spectrum with what was formerly called Asperger's Syndrome. None disagreed, but all stated that the treatment would be the same. Our family longs for the day that the treatments will be specific for the area of the brain responsible for each symptom a person has.

Mary has an appreciation for Robert's brain-based suffering. Although she has never had a psychotic experience, she knows first-hand what brain-based suffering is like. Her exact words were, "Mom, most people think that no matter what else happens, they will be able to control their minds. What they don't realize is that a mind does not always act in a person's best interest." Even more incredible was the day that she said to me, "Mom, I cannot tell you how awful this is. All you can think about is escaping! If someone offered you something that made you think it might help, you would try it. Mom, you would not ask is it good for me. Will it work? Is it legal? Oh, Mom, you would just do it hoping to escape." I was hearing my daughter who was valedictorian of her class, junior prom queen and president of student government as she shared with me the reality of life from her perspective.

Mary Becomes Dr. Comer

Another memory is from 1995 when Mary received her hood for completing her Ph.D. in Electrical Engineering at Purdue. Mary's husband, Steve Comer, handed me a copy of her dissertation after the ceremony. I did not read it until we returned home. The first page reads:

MULTIRESOLUTION IMAGE PROCESSING
TECHNIQUES WITH
APPLICATIONS IN TEXTURE SEGMENTATION
AND NONLINEAR FILTERING

A Thesis
Submitted to the Faculty
of
Purdue University
by
Mary L. Comer
In Partial Fulfillment of the
Requirements for the Degree
of
Doctor of Philosophy
December 1995

The next page reads:

To my brother Robert, who has taught me the most important lessons in life.

I took the dissertation down the hall to Robert's bedroom and pointed to that page. He read those words silently. Tears streamed down his cheeks.

Chapter 14

Back Home to Hagerstown

The ongoing challenge for Robert at Burris was the travel. The special-ed teacher said he was just too tired. She made several trips to Hagerstown. The cooperative at that time made no provisions for high-school students to be served in Hagerstown. Robert had finished the 8th, 9th, and 10th grades at Burris. He would be coming back to Hagerstown High School for his junior and senior years. The special-ed teacher explained to the assembled administrators that it would not be appropriate to put Robert on a school bus to Laurel, Indiana for the special-ed classroom there because that would pose even a greater transportation problem than he had at Burris. She argued that the travel made him too tired to learn.

The special-ed teacher at Burris who came to Hagerstown to plead on Robert's behalf won. I recall the head of the cooperative that served students in need of services at the time as saying, "If I provide services at Hagerstown High School, do you know how many students that will be?" I answered that I did not know. He said, "One." I replied, "Yes, and that one is my son."

Robert was happy to be back home for his junior year in school. He had made friends at Burris and continued to visit them on occasion, but he had kept up with friends at home. He was able to work at Ralph's office or drive to New Castle to make deliveries for Ralph. His junior year at school went well. He was mainstreamed, but the cooperative provided an itinerant special education teacher who negotiated with Robert's teachers to accommodate him in the regular classroom.

The cooperative required her to work with him on Tuesdays, which was not helpful to him because he needed her help at the end of the week to prepare for the week ahead. We worked with him at home more than was good for him. Sending a student who has special needs to school during regular school hours and making him do even more than the usual homework plus household chores is less than ideal. But we made it work! Robert graduated with his class.

Chapter 15

We Enter the World of Mental Illness

It was 1981 and the beginning of his senior year. Robert was eighteen years old. He had asked to go to a religious retreat with a friend. It only occurred to me in retrospect how strange it was that he did not have to take pajamas. They had instructed that those attending would not need night clothes. He left on a Friday night and looked forward only to having a good time.

The Accident

As a defense attorney, Ralph frequently had nighttime calls, so he was the one who answered the phone in the middle of that Friday night. I heard him ask if the matter could wait until morning. Then he hung up and told me Robert needed to be picked up because Robert said that they were scaring the hell out of him. I heard the car leave as Ralph went in the early hours of the morning toward Indianapolis, which was about sixty miles away, in addition to some miles south to the place where the retreat was being held.

As I learned later, Robert had left the retreat grounds and gone to a farmhouse not too far away to ask to use the phone. What had frightened Robert so badly? The church holding the retreat was a different Protestant faith from ours. They kept the teenagers up all night and were telling them how important it was to be "sanctified."

Robert told them he did not know what they were talking about. He said that although he attended church every week and went to vacation Bible school, he did not know what being sanctified meant and his parents were not sanctified. They responded by informing him that without being sanctified, he and his parents would go to hell. Robert left. He walked to a nearby farmhouse where someone opened the door to a small terrified teenager who asked to use the telephone. Ralph picked him up and calmed him as best he could before they started the hundred mile or so trip home.

On the way the yellow Ford Fiesta they were driving was suddenly hit from behind. Ralph later told me how eerie an experience it was. He lost control of the car. It veered across the centerline and collided with another car (T-bone). An irate nineteen-year-old man jumped out and shouted that Ralph was in his lane. Ralph replied that he had not put himself there. Robert was not wearing a seatbelt (it was before there were seatbelt laws). Ralph was wearing his, but he still had a bump on his forehead. Robert banged his head against the dash and flew backward into the back seat. He had a large bump on his forehead and a scraped back to show for it. Robert said that he had seen a car veer across the road and disappear down an embankment. So, they all three ran to the side of the road and looked down into a space where there was a car upside down with no driver. Ralph told me later he could not imagine how anyone could have survived such an accident and then run away.

Ralph said over and over, "Joan, it was so unreal." I found out that all of this had happened when at 4:00 a.m. I got a phone call from Robert. "Mom, Dad and I are okay, but you will need to pick us up because we have been in an accident and Dad cannot drive the car. There is too much damage." I drove to the hospital he was calling from on the far south side of Indianapolis to pick them up. The yellow Ford Fiesta was totaled.

The Break

Robert had problems over the next week or so. I could tell he was struggling but he kept on going. Then one day when I returned from my work in Indianapolis, I found my younger daughters weeping. Robert was in the hospital and Dad was there with him. I headed to Richmond to find that Robert had been admitted to the psychiatric unit. He was out of control and out of touch.

It was about ten days after the accident. The brain, nervous, and endocrine systems, as well as the interactions between them, are complex and even today not well-understood. Suddenly our family entered the world of those brain-based illnesses we call mental illnesses. Through the years he took the anticholinergic medication faithfully. It kept many of the symptoms at bay, but it could not make the voices go away. They were voices that he heard but were silent to the rest of us.

Robert was in the psychiatric unit for about a month when the psychiatrist went into his room and told him that he was going home on furlough. All Robert heard was that he was going home. "Furlough" meant nothing to him. Once he was at home, he refused to go back.

In the meantime, I was dealing with unpleasant issues of my own. Ralph had been with Robert when he had his break with reality. He took him to Richmond from our home in Hagerstown. They first went to the community mental health center in Richmond. The Medical Director at that time knew that Robert was having a psychotic break, but he acknowledged that there were newer medications than he was using, and he knew of a private psychiatrist who used them. He referred Ralph to him, and he was the one who had Robert hospitalized.

When I got to the hospital that evening, it was still visiting hours. The attendant took me through several locked doors to Robert, who was alone in a small, bare room. I remember so little of that visit. What I can remember is that Robert's neck was twisted at an odd angle. I learned later that was a side effect of one of the medications he was given. He was frantic and complaining about hearing many different voices that seemed to be harassing him unmercifully. I also remember that Robert was surrounded by cigarette butts and had a pack of cigarettes with only a few remaining. Although he may have smoked occasionally before, like so many people with a diagnosis of schizophrenia, he became a chain smoker. Several years later, a bout of bronchitis caused him to stop cold turkey.

Schizophrenogenic Mom

Although I had seen Robert the night before, I did not visit with the psychiatrist until the next day. The psychiatrist's first words to me were that my son heard voices. I replied that I was aware of that. The psychiatrist asked me whether I knew whose voice my son heard. I knew that Robert had heard the voices of Jesus Christ, Adolf Hitler, and others. The psychiatrist gave me another answer: "My mother." The psychiatrist asked me why I thought Robert would say that it was his mother's voice.

I thought at first that he might be joking with me. The answer that came to my mind was that Robert was ill. The psychiatrist made it very clear in the next few moments that he was not joking. This was a very serious matter, and if I had been the mother I should have been, he would not be treating my son.

I was stunned. I knew what he was saying was not true because I was teaching the physiological facts regarding brain and behavior at the time. At that moment I made a promise to myself that I would see that mothers did not receive that message. As mothers we accept responsibility for everything our children do, so many moms would buy right into that message. How damaging! It was not that I was a perfect mother. I made mistakes on a regular basis, but I knew that these were symptoms of an illness I had not caused.

It was obvious that the nurses believed I had caused the illness, and the meeting with the social worker began with her questioning me. I was carrying my briefcase, which prompted her to ask, "Do you always carry your work with you?" I was not sure of her implications, but I knew they were not supportive of me as a mom.

Robert became ill at a time when students in most health-care programs were still being taught that the cause of schizophrenia was faulty family dynamics. The person who was scrutinized the most was the mother. For that reason, the term "Schizophrenogenic Mom" labeled the mother as the one responsible for giving rise to (or causing) schizophrenia. Studies of mothers interacting with adult children who had been diagnosed with schizophrenia only made matters worse. If an adult child has schizophrenia the mother will, of course, interact differently, but the interaction is reactionary rather than causal.

Today we have shifted more toward understanding mental illnesses as being brain-based illnesses with behavioral symptoms. Even more significant is the fact that students in all areas of health care are learning the value of applying behavioral health care across the gamut of body systems. I sense that health-care programs are teaching more holistic care. I consider that a sign of progress.

Two organizations have been instrumental in bringing that change. An organization now named NAMI was formed in Madison, Wisconsin in 1979 by family members who had been blamed for their adult children's schizophrenia. When the Indiana Alliance for the Mentally Ill, now known as The National Alliance on Mental Illness-Indiana (NAMI Indiana), formed in 1985, our family became charter members. Robert loved attending meetings and made friends with other members and their families.

Ralph and I also became active in the Mental Health Association, now called Mental Health America (MHA). MHA has the wider scope of Mental Health and NAMI focuses on

Mental Illnesses. Both organizations recognize the importance of education. Ralph, Robert and I began attending state and national conferences of NAMI where we heard medical experts talk on brain studies and new treatments as they were developed.

Robert had a goal of graduating from high school. He had even investigated the possibility of attending Vincennes College. He used his first phone call from the psychiatric ward to call the Hagerstown High School principal to make sure he could still graduate. He did graduate with his class. First, the school provided a teacher who came to the house and became a special friend. Then he was slowly re-introduced to the classes he needed to graduate. The school and the teachers made every effort to support him and us as a family.

Chapter 16

Dr. Dunlop's Answer to Robert's Question

R alph made the decision that the hospital in Richmond was unable to meet Robert's needs well enough. There was limited space to serve a wide range of people. It was a sad decision for Ralph because it would put more distance between him and his son. He prolonged making it. At the time I was a postdoctoral fellow at Riley Children's Hospital in Indianapolis. A colleague arranged an appointment at Riley with a pediatric psychiatrist down the hall from our clinic and research lab.

Robert Was Admitted to an Adult Psychiatric Unit at University Hospital

The pediatric psychiatrist did some testing and discussed the situation with me. I recall distinctly that he said Robert must have been a pretty good age before he could tie his shoes. I smiled remembering Robert's request for help with that. The psychiatrist also discussed having Robert admitted immediately to an adult unit at University Hospital because he was over 18. He was a close friend of the director of that unit and decided to have Robert admitted that day for evaluation and a medication change.

It was Robert's twentieth birthday. I asked whether I could take Robert to a restaurant for a birthday dinner before admitting him at University Hospital. It is interesting to note how many birthdays after his psychotic break that Robert was hospitalized. After dinner when I brought Robert back to be admitted, I could stay for a while.

I remember there was a woman who asked him questions about the voices that he heard. She asked whether they were loud or soft, friendly, unfriendly, or both. As he answered her questions calmly and factually, I felt as if I were eavesdropping on a conversation I was not meant to hear. How could my beloved son be carrying on a conversation that seemed rational, but sounded so irrational to me? I saw him to his room and said good-bye with a promise to visit. He was in my territory now.

I don't remember how long he was in the psychiatric unit at University Hospital or exactly what medication changes they made, but he did improve. One psychiatry resident connected very well with Robert and seemed to enjoy visiting with me when I came to see Robert. When it was time for Robert to be discharged, he explained that he was not able to treat Robert after he left the hospital, but the attending psychiatrist, Dr. Stephen Dunlop, had agreed to treat him if that was what my husband and I wanted.

I remembered Dr. Dunlop as the psychiatrist who had spoken with me about Robert's medication change. He had said, "You and your husband are different from many parents we see. You don't seem to blame either Robert or yourselves for his illness." He added that often he had to spend a lot of time explaining to parents that they had not caused the illness. I smiled and nodded. There would be no useful purpose in my telling him about my experience just two years earlier of being blamed by a very competent psychiatrist for Robert's illness. I also knew that the psychiatrist was no longer giving that message to mothers because I checked with families through NAMI.

I remember distinctly our first visit to Dr. Dunlop's office, which was on the second floor of a barracks building on the grounds of the Indiana University School of Medicine. The barracks had been constructed on the campus either before or during World War II for some reason and were then relegated to the Department of Psychiatry as office space. I remember climbing the creaking wooden steps and listening to Robert's question, "Mom, what is happening to me? What is happening to my mind?" I didn't tell him that his dad and I were pondering the same question. I answered, "I think that is a wonderful question for you to ask your new psychiatrist."

Soon we were seated in the small room that served as Dr. Dunlop's office. It barely held the chairs we were sitting on, and a rather large desk where Dr. Dunlop was seated across from us. Robert remembered, "What is happening to me? What is happening to my mind?"

Dr. Dunlop paused. He was silent for what seemed like a long time as if to consider exactly how to answer such a curious question. "Well, Robert, your mind plays tricks on you because you have an illness. It isn't a new illness, people all over the world have had the same illness that you do for centuries. The good news is that now we have medicine to treat it. That's why you were in the hospital, so you could get adjusted to the new medicines we started you on."

Robert must have asked him what he meant by saying his mind played tricks on him. I don't remember. What I do remember is Dr. Dunlop's response. "Robert, if I leave the room believing that I have left this pencil holder here and come back into the room and the pencil holder is over there, my mind allows me all kinds of possibilities. I can think to myself that I must have been mistaken about where I left the pencil holder. My mind allows me to think that someone must have come in when I was out of the room and moved the pencil holder from here to there. Your mind plays a trick on you by making you think that the pencil holder moved itself and we all know that pencil holders do not have muscles, so they cannot move themselves."

As I pondered all that he had said, I took time to notice that the pencil holder he was moving from place to place appeared to be a gift made from a jar or can covered with paper or felt. Perhaps it was a gift from one of his children. I also took time to remember that Robert must have shared in the hospital that he saw trees in a neighbor's yard that moved farther down the street the next day. After I worked through all of that, I had a more startling revelation. Dr. Dunlop's explanation had taken away my fear of Robert's illness.

Chapter 17

I Am a Classy Mom

I have friends and colleagues who keep diaries or journals. If I keep track of time and place it is only by connecting those within a structure I can remember. For example, I can tell you the year each one of my children was born. To tell you her or his age at any given time, I need to do the math. Why? I believe it has to do with my enjoying the flow of life within boundaries.

My memories of those years that Robert lived and was treated in Indianapolis are like that. The stream of events flowed like a river that bends and curves, crashing over the rocks along the way. Regarding life with Robert, I remember the twists and turns and crashing over rocks much easier than the times of an even flow along the straight ways.

Introduction to the Code Word

I remember well that Dr. Dunlop moved from the Medical Center to establish a practice and direct a program at a hospital south of Indianapolis. I remember that Robert had times that he functioned better than others. He was admitted to the hospital several times. It was here that we first encountered the code word.

I was the only person who could call to ask about how Robert was doing. Before anyone on that unit would speak to me, I had to give my name and give them the code word. At this hospital psychiatric and addictions patients were crowded together. Patients in that unit were not acknowledged as patients in that hospital. If friends sent cards, they were returned to sender marked, "not at this address."

How I hated having to use a code word. I remember reading a short story years ago by a mother of a ten-year-old disabled girl who was being bullied on her way to school. In those days there were no special education programs to meet the girl's needs. She and her husband realized that their only option was to send their beloved daughter to a residential home a considerable distance from where they lived. The mom's instructions were to sew her daughter's code into all her personal possessions such as her clothes and items she brought with her, including her toys. Her daughter carefully picked the toys. Among them was her doll, Maribelle. The mother commented on seeing the doll with the code prominently displayed on her leg. The mother wrote that she thought that the doll did not like the code word very much. Maribelle was a very classy doll. Robert was in and out of several behavioral health units that required a code word. Each time I was forced to use it, I reminded myself that I am a very classy mom.

Let me explain here that my objection was not that a code-word system was used. My objection was that there was no patient choice on this matter. Traditionally, patients on all units except Behavioral Health must petition to have their presence in the hospital remain unlisted. Patients in Behavioral Health units have no choice but are automatically assigned to the code list and therefore, do not exist as patients in that hospital.

When someone called who was not the designated representative and owner of the code word for that patient, the operator response was, "There is no patient in this hospital by that name." A patient who was admitted to the hospital for any reason should have had the option to be on the code-word/

hospital patient list. The default could have been that all patients were on that list until they chose to be taken off.

Some categories of people were put on the list automatically. Behavioral Health was at the top of the list. If the practice were adjusted as I suggest above, the stigma would be lessened. Another restriction on the Behavioral Health unit that did not apply to many other units was limited visiting hours. The reason given for this was that group sessions were held for these patients. The assumption was that group sessions were particularly beneficial only for those with Behavioral Health issues.

Group sessions might be beneficial for any patient in the hospital. The emphasis on group sessions for behavioral health patients is that these disorders are behavioral-based rather than brain-based. Why would a person with a brain-based disorder be any more helped by a group session than a person with heart failure or breast cancer? Many persons who have one of the brain-based disorders are helped more by one-on-one counseling sessions than participating in group therapy. That is not an anti-group statement at all. Some patients benefit greatly from group therapy; others may benefit from one-on-one counseling; and still others from other forms of treatment. Certainly, restricting visiting hours to three hours a day because of the need for group sessions is extreme.

Another problem with the limited visiting hours is the consequence of removing family and other loved ones' care from the doctor-patient interview, or indeed, any interview with the psychiatrist. This consequence is often costly. We need to abandon behavioral health as a term describing brain-based illness. All illnesses have a behavioral component. There is nothing more behavioral than a heart attack. The person exhibits very bizarre behavior. That behavior identifies what is happening, but we don't use the term behavioral health when a person exhibits the symptoms of a heart attack. That term is reserved only to refer to patients with psychiatric disorders. It is complicated enough for any patient, but with the additional restrictions for Behavioral Health patients, the system becomes almost impossible to manage. It is a splintered system whose patients may already be struggling with confusion.

I remember when Ralph had a blocked carotid artery that finally caused a stroke-like response until the doctors performed an endarterectomy to clear the artery. The doctor said to me, "We need you. We can see what your husband is like now. What we need to find out is what he was like before this happened. How has he changed?"

I pondered why these same kinds of conversations often do not occur between doctors and families when the patient is in a behavioral-health unit. One reason may be a remnant from the time when faulty family dynamics was considered the cause of mental illnesses. Another reason might be that many behavioral-health units have limited hours that family can visit. The opportunity for family to be present while doctors are making their rounds is not as likely to occur.

Behavioral Health practices can limit accountability. For example, I receive surveys from our university health system for all other conditions for which all members of our family have been treated. These surveys provide an opportunity for patient and family to give feedback to the unit. On the other hand, I never received a survey for Robert for any of his experiences in behavioral health. I asked the social worker why recently. Her answer dealt with confidentiality issues.

Certainly, hospitals need to practice confidentiality, but sometimes it seems extreme in the behavioral-health system. I experienced this firsthand after Robert had been a patient in a Behavioral Health unit. I sent a greeting in December addressed to the director who had been especially kind and helpful. It was returned months later in April in an envelope that was completely void of any trace of where it had been. The new envelope had only my name and address. I was surprised not only by the delay but also by the extreme effort to keep the behavioral-health unit confidential even though I was the one who had addressed it to Behavioral Health in the first place.

Several hospitals have tried ways to get around the stigma of the code word, but their follow-through is poor. Some hospitals require every patient or family to choose a code word regardless of the reason the person is hospitalized. At one facility we asked why we needed a code word for Robert. We were assured that all patients regardless of the nature of the hospitalization needed a code word. They never asked us for the code word after that because it was not a behavioral-health issue. He had been admitted for a bowel prep. A friend whose wife was admitted to that same unit said they had to choose a code word but were never asked for it again.

Chapter 18

Robert's Wanderings

Robert had a way of disappearing no matter how closely we monitored him. It wasn't that he ran away, he simply wandered off and would be lost. On one weekend night we celebrated a family event in the Union Station in downtown Indianapolis. Even though we had a dozen people in our group, Robert managed to wander away. In my mind I pictured him wandering out of the building and being lost on the streets of downtown Indy. We split into groups and finally one group found him. When I saw that he was safe, I cried. Every time after that when he wandered away, after we found him, he'd say, "Mom, you aren't going to cry, are you?"

Finally, Dr. Dunlop told us that he had come to the limit of his ability to treat Robert. I knew that his expertise was in treating mood disorders. He suggested that we investigate having Robert admitted to Larue Carter Memorial Hospital, a state hospital near the IU Medical Center in Indianapolis. He suggested a specific psychiatrist who had success treating patients diagnosed with refractory schizophrenia. There was a wait time of about a month.

To say it was a challenging month is a terrific understatement. I remember taking Robert to a national NAMI convention in San Antonio, Texas. Ralph, Robert and I stayed in a hotel across from the Alamo. Robert disappeared at the Alamo.

The good news is that the Alamo was covered by police who were on foot, horseback, bicycle, and automobile. They found Robert, and the whole Indiana contingency kept a very close eye on him for the rest of the national conference.

Chapter 19

Larue Carter Memorial Hospital

Finally, we received a call that there was a place for him at Larue Carter Hospital. The first hospitalization was at the Larue Carter Hospital that was then on West 10th Street on the edge of the IU School of Medicine campus. It was a crowded facility. Robert was in a unit on the first floor that had rooms for men on one end and for women on the other, with a large common day room in between.

Memories of that experience are buried deep inside because it was so difficult for me. Larue Carter had many advantages over Central State Hospital that was about two miles west. Central State was a long-term care hospital whose residents had little hope for recovery. Larue Carter was established for intermediate care with many of its patients involved in transla-tional research. That meant that the psychiatrists had access to experimental medications and treatment programs. The social worker that we were assigned told me that the psychiatrist Dr. Dunlop had recommended did not meet with family members. A NAMI friend found a psychiatrist who had retired from Central State Hospital and worked part time as a consultant at Larue Carter. He agreed to meet and discuss Robert's treatment with us. I will always be grateful to him for keeping me informed during a very difficult time.

Our social worker at Larue Carter was wonderful. He could help me understand Robert's socialization progress and assisted with informing me about possible next steps. He told me when Robert was ready to go from Carter to a partial hospitalization program a few buildings away. The goal was to prepare him for release from the hospital to return home.

One afternoon I received a call from the social worker informing me that he was going to have to put an all-points bulletin out on Robert because he had not returned from partial hospitalization. Robert had been under such close supervision at the hospital that the social worker was unaware of his tendency to wander. I explained that Robert may have gotten confused and lost, but I could not believe that he had intentionally "escaped." That gave the social worker an idea. He went to the person who was supposed to bring Robert back to Carter. That person had forgotten Robert and told the social worker where Robert was supposed to wait.

The next call from the social worker brought a sigh of relief. Robert was still sitting there, waiting to be picked up. The social worker said with a laugh, that of all the people involved, Robert was the one who did exactly what he was supposed to do. After his discharge from Larue Carter Hospital he continued with the partial hospitalization program and was treated as an outpatient at Carter.

When it became necessary for him to be admitted to Larue Carter again, the hospital had moved to a vacated VA hospital on Cold Springs Road in Indianapolis. The spacious building and even more spacious grounds were much more appropriate for residents. At this new location, I was able to serve on several committees and boards.

When the psychiatrist who had served as a liaison to explain Robert's medical treatment to me retired fully, my NAMI friend attempted to find someone to replace him. The hospital superintendent was appreciative of my volunteer service to the hospital. She said that she would find a psychiatrist to fill that role.

A few days later, I received a call from the then Medical Director of Adult Psychiatric Services, Dr. Jeffrey Kellams. He read me a list of psychiatrists and a brief profile of each. Then he added that he would also be happy to fill that role. I accepted his invitation. Dr. Kellams has remained in our lives as a friend and off and on as an important part of Robert's treatment, as both Dr. Kellams and Robert moved from one program to another. He has remained a colleague and friend after Robert's death. I will always be grateful to Dr. Kellams for the time and concern he has dedicated to our family.

Chapter 20

Riverpointe

Robert and I commuted to Indianapolis from Hagerstown most days beginning when his psychiatric care moved to Indianapolis and lasted for a little over four years. When Dr. Baehner moved to Children's Hospital of Los Angeles, I became a Research Associate in Pediatric Hematology Oncology at Riley Hospital and remained as an assistant Professor part time in the Physiology Department at the School of Medicine. It was a good time for Robert. The medications allowed him to function as well as possible, and he made many friends around Riley Hospital and other hospitals on the School of Medicine campus and the surrounding neighborhood.

He was no longer driving a car. One day Dr. Dunlop left a voice message on my answering machine. I heard him say, "I am no longer comfortable having Robert driving a car." I thought at the time that Dr. Dunlop may have gone to a conference where they had cautioned psychiatrists about legal considerations if they had not expressed some concern. I wrote a note to Dr. Dunlop informing him that I had read his message of concern regarding Robert's driving. My thinking was that it would give him written documentation. Then I rode as a passenger when Robert was driving. He did a great job.

I was surprised one day three or four weeks later when Robert informed me that he wasn't going to drive anymore. I was more than surprised. I was stunned. He loved to drive. It caused me to reconsider the motive behind Dr. Dunlop's call. What had he noticed that I missed? I never asked and neither the doctor nor Robert told me.

In August of 1987 I accepted a teaching position at Indiana University East (IU East) in Richmond. Earlier that year the Board of Trustees had established a Bachelor of Science degree in Biology for that campus. I responded to an advertisement for someone to teach Anatomy and Physiology to nursing and allied health sciences students. When I accepted the position, the Interim Chancellor asked whether I would be able to keep my research at the School of Medicine in Indianapolis because at that time IU East had no research facilities for faculty research. By that time all three of our daughters were in college. Ralph, Robert and I made it work. Compared to the challenges of graduate school and providing transportation to Burris, it was a breeze.

I was promoted and tenured in 1994 and granted a sabbatical leave. I was able to rent an apartment in Indianapolis at a high-rise building called Riverpointe close to campus. Many graduate students lived there and Riverpointe provided a shuttle service to the university and back. Robert loved Riverpointe. Several times a week Ralph commuted to eat dinner at Riley and spend the night at Riverpointe. Robert and I went home Saturday afternoon and stayed through Sunday.

Chapter 21

Welcome to Robert's House

E ven though Robert had up times and down times that included hospitalizations, he was so happy at Riverpointe that when we saw an area was opening in a small neighborhood very near to the School of Medicine, Ralph and I stopped by the rental office.

Ransom Place

This neighborhood was three city blocks east to west and two city blocks south to north. Before and during the civil war people of color moved from the southern United States north. Many felt that by the time they were midway up in Indiana they were safe enough to settle in cities like Richmond, Fountain City, and Indianapolis. Many came via the Underground Railroad and were supported by members of the Society of Friends (Quakers) along the way. A Quaker, Levi Coffin, provided a station on the Underground Railroad in Fountain City, Indiana. There is still a museum bearing his name.

Some came to Indianapolis and moved into the area that was occupied at that time by working class Irish who had come to Indianapolis from Baltimore, Maryland. The Irish/Baltimore influence lingers with streets named Paca and St. Clair. That small six-block area became Ransom Place. It was named for Freeman Ransom who was the attorney for Madam Walker, a woman of color who had begun as a laundress, then was a hairdresser and created an empire by developing special hair products for African American women.

Paca Street

The houses along the two blocks of Paca Street and some of the condemned houses back in the neighborhood were razed before remaining residents had the rest of the neighborhood declared historic. We purchased a lot on Paca Street and as the construction began, we stopped by to watch the house go up. Some of the residents came from back in the neighborhood to welcome us. I remember the gratitude we felt at being accepted as ones who were "different" moving in.

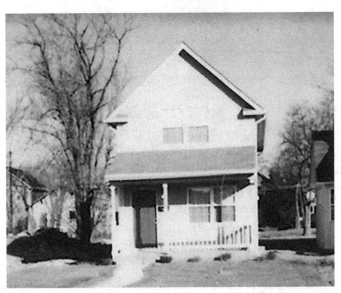

Robert's home on Paca St. under construction

A small sign over the door leading to the dining area greeted the world, Welcome to Robert's House. He chose the color of the siding and made other choices as they became available. He was the first inhabitant of the new "Paca Street." He could walk the neighborhood. Several restaurants opened in the commercial area across the street. With some telephone calls in the morning and evening, Ralph and I could leave him overnight. He was compliant with medication and managed well. The longest he stayed by himself was two nights.

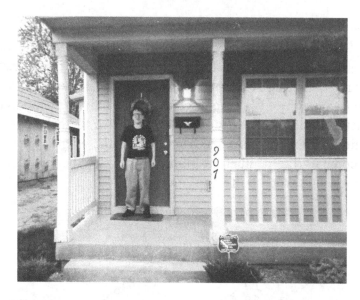

Over the years Robert lived in his house on Paca Street, schizophrenia and the treatments for it took more and more of him. Finally, we could no longer leave him on his own at night. Eventually we had to keep him under continuous surveillance. I remember, sadly, the day he was upset with me for a reason I do not recall. He stalked out of the front door and down the walk to the public sidewalk and turned.

Through the front window, I watched him go. I did not try to call to him or stop him in any way. I remembered that years ago before he was ill, Ralph and I promised each other we would never hold him back or hold him so close that he could not make his own decisions. I saw him slow his pace and stop. I cannot remember how long he thought it over, but it seemed forever. Then he turned around and slowly retraced his steps. I left the front room before he reopened the front door and came back in his house. Although he continued to wander, never again did he intentionally leave. For me it marked the day that Robert faced the sad reality of his dependence on us and his trust that we would keep him safe.

I was reassured by his ability to make decisions in his own best interest. Through the years of psychoses and degeneration of his abilities, he continued to have some moments of self-preservation and unclouded decision-making. Today, as difficult as it is to accept his death, I feel a tinge of joy in knowing that schizophrenia could not rob him of everything.

Rusty Saves Us

My new neighbor, Sylva, stood at my bedside at 2:00 one morning and calmly told me that my adult son, Robert, was on her front porch. She explained that she was certain that Robert had not rung the bell, or she would have heard it, but her dog, Rusty, persisted, and his barking prompted her to go to the door to investigate.

All I could think was that this nightmare was real. When it dawned on Sylva that I was experiencing shell shock, she retrieved Robert from her front porch and carefully led him back through the door he had left wide-open as he wandered out into the dark, silent night. He must have been confused about which sidewalk to choose to get him back to safety. Her mission completed, Sylva left me to watch Robert closely through the night. This was a new development in my relationship with Robert. The next morning, I joined the fellowship of families with loved ones who wander. We had to install locks and chains that lock with a key for all doors that led to the outside of the house.

The next evening, I heard Rusty bark again, and I spoke to him aloud from my chair, "Hi, Rusty dear friend. Thank you for saving us from disaster. How are you doing, Dear One?" Overnight, Rusty changed my anti-canine attitude toward barking dogs. Even more humbling was licking the crumbs of my long-held belief that the most difficult and drawn out process in the world is changing an attitude.

8C Methodist

It will help you, the reader, understand what it took me several years to find out about the C building at the Methodist Hospital in Indianapolis. It is a different hospital from the rest of the medical Methodist Hospital. It is the Behavioral Health Hospital. A person needed to be admitted to Behavioral Health Methodist regardless of their previous location. Some came from home, others from another hospital, some were under arrest but had probable "behavioral-health" issues. Even those patients who had been in the emergency room or a medical unit at the Methodist Hospital had to be discharged from Methodist Hospital before they could be admitted to Methodist Behavioral Health for psychiatric care.

Weekends were the worst when Robert was on 8C at the Methodist Hospital. Visiting hours for family were limited to 12:00 to 1:00 and 4:00 to 6:00 in the afternoon, as I recall. Staff psychiatrists tended to make rounds according to the head psychiatrist's schedule. That was usually in the morning before visiting hours for family or others who had the secret code word (and that number was limited). Family members laughed because when the person at the desk came out to get the code word anyone could hear all other patient's code words. Perhaps it was irony and stress that forced us to find humor in any situation.

Electroconvulsive Therapy (ECT)

ECT has evolved from findings centuries ago that seizures helped alleviate the symptoms of psychosis. In the late 1930's psychiatrists in Italy used electricity to provoke the seizures. ECT became a very controversial form of treatment in mental hospitals in many countries. Part of the controversy was that it was performed on patients who were awake and often suffered side effects or injuries that were not worth any benefit that they received. Although the procedure has been revised with the use of anesthesia and muscle relaxants, memory loss remains a problem. It has become a method of choice for women who are pregnant, especially those who are severely depressed and/ or suicidal. It is also used for patients with severe psychoses who are resistant to other therapies.

Robert has done well with ECT treatments that began when he was at Larue Carter Hospital and continued for more than twenty years at the Methodist Behavioral Health. Mid-February in 2019, the policy for administering ECTs changed, so the last two for Robert were performed in the cardiology unit of Methodist Hospital.

Chapter 22

The Need for Integrated Treatment of Mental Illness and Addictions

Robert and our friends in NAMI taught our family that there is a strong connection between mental illness and addiction. People with a diagnosis of a psychiatric disorder and families with a loved-one with such a diagnosis shared their stories with us. Their illnesses covered the spectrum of mental illnesses. A common theme among them was the fact that the symptoms in each case first appeared between the ages of twelve and eighteen. According to the NAMI website over half of adult persons with a drug-use disorder have a co-occurring mental illness.

Robert's co-occurring issue involved schizophrenia and cigarettes. I mentioned earlier in this book about the many cigarette butts I noticed the first night of his psychotic break. In fact, he developed a minimum three-pack-a-day need to smoke, until a bout of bronchitis forced him to quit. Later I learned from friends at NAMI that it is common for persons with schizophrenia to begin smoking cigarettes or to increase that habit.

Schizophrenia occurs in about 1% of the population worldwide. The occurrence increases to 40% in identical twins. That fact indicates there is a genetic component to schizophrenia.

However, the brain is so complex that understanding the details of genetic contributions to co-occurring addictions and mental illnesses will require more research.

Dr. R. A. (Andy) Chambers is the Director of Addiction Psychiatry Training at Indiana University School of Medicine in Indianapolis. Dr. Chambers used animal models in his research of mental illness and addiction. By destroying different portions of the brain, he was able to test for the effects of several mental illnesses. He was also able to test the effects of different addictive substances at the same time. These studies led him to develop the 2 × 4 Model.

I had received an Indiana University intercampus grant earlier in Dr. Chambers' career which allowed me to collaborate with researchers in his lab. My small portion of the research that led to his development of the 2 × 4 Model limited my understanding of the entire model. Recently, Dr. Chambers explained more about the model to me. It is about the fact that a person who has a mental illness is more vulnerable to addiction as well as being more vulnerable to an increased severity of addiction. Separating the care for persons who have a diagnosis of mental illness without treating the addiction concurrently is not scientifically valid.

Dr. Chambers' work provides the brain-based science of the model. He identifies the brain structure that is responsible for motivational programming under the influence of input from other brain structures that he names specifically. The problem arises when the professional people, who treat persons who are mentally ill, do not understand and ignore treating their addictions at the same time. Addiction is a grieving process involving loss. Health care providers who do not understand the process involving relapses, and the hard work involved in recovery, can often do more harm than good. For readers who wish to learn more, an article Dr. Chambers co-authored is listed in the reference section at the end of this book.

The 2 × 4 Model is the foundation of a clinical plan that provides integrated treatment for people who have one or more mental illnesses and are also addicted to at least one substance of abuse. According to Dr. Chambers, a Venn diagram that shows a circle representing all persons with a diagnosis of one or more mental illnesses, intersecting with another circle representing all people who have an addiction of any kind, has an area of overlap that represents those who have a diagnosis of both. That overlapping area represents roughly 50 to 60% of the total. In his book titled, *The 2 × 4 Model*, he describes a blueprint for a possible nation-wide system of integrated addiction and mental health treatment.

Chapter 23

The Difference Between a Broken Brain and a Blocked Bowel

Robert's cousin Brad died unexpectedly May 4, 2016. His sudden death was traumatic for Robert. At that time his sister Leanne was taking Robert for his ECT treatments at the C building. Both Leanne and the ECT staff were very much concerned about Robert's extreme withdrawal, almost catatonic condition. Leanne cancelled her appointments for the day and waited with Robert until he was admitted to 8C. Once she was given his room number, and the code word had been established, she called me with the details. We agreed that I could go visit him before visiting hours ended at 6:00 p.m.

I was sitting outside the hospital calling the switchboard operator who said, "We have no patient in the hospital by that name." I pressed, "But I know he is there. My daughter sat all day in the emergency room while he was admitted. He is on the eighth floor and the code word is Yoko Ono." The operator repeated, "We have no patient by that name." I pressed further. "What should I do? You have lost my son!" The operator replied, "You will need to check other hospitals in the city to see if he is a patient there."

I hung up the phone and left a message on my son-in-law's message machine, "Brent and Leanne, the Methodist Hospital has lost Robert. What do you suggest I do?" An hour or so later Leanne called, "Mom we listened to your message. We laughed because you were so calm. You very calmly informed us that the hospital had lost Robert. I suggest you call the floor directly. I did not give you that number before." I called and the nurse assured me that Robert was there.

Monday morning the psychiatrist called me. He was concerned because Robert had complained of shortness of breath, so that psychiatrist ordered an electrocardiogram. He was concerned because the test results indicated Robert might have a coronary blockage.

The doctor then ordered an echocardiogram for that afternoon and told me he would move Robert from 8C (Behavioral Health) to 8B (a medical surgery unit that was reserved for psychiatric patients who needed medical attention). 8B had regular visiting hours for family, but I still needed the hated code word. I smiled again at the irony of his comment because I considered psychiatric issues the same as medical.

That afternoon I met Robert on 8B. I noticed that his tummy, which was always large, resembled the abdominal size of an average pregnant woman who was approximately halfway through her pregnancy. I was permitted to go to the unit where they did the echocardiogram. The gentleman in charge of greeting patients and families assured me that Robert was being evaluated by the topnotch cardiologist because the psychiatrist had indicated how special Robert was. The cardiologist explained the procedure to me. He would use Robert's femoral artery to thread the line, and he would be able to examine all of Robert's heart function and take a picture of his heart. When the procedure was finished the cardiologist assured me that Robert's heart was in great shape. He could not have a healthier heart. I accompanied Robert back to 8B where he had been admitted, but I knew something was terribly wrong. His tummy had expanded to the size greater than any pregnant woman I had ever seen.

The psychiatrist came in to tell me the good news about the echocardiogram study. He took one look at Robert's tummy. I saw the terror in his eyes before he disappeared. Later I learned that he had made a frantic emergency call to the family-practice unit right across the street from the Methodist Hospital.

The next thing I knew a doctor I had never met came rushing through Robert's door. The psychiatrist introduced him quickly. I learned later he retired a year after our meeting. The fact that he had rushed was obvious. He was perspiring and breathless. I was amazed at how quickly a man of such advanced age could get there. He said that Robert was going to be moved to the 4th floor, which was a medical surgery unit with multiple monitoring capabilities. He left the room to place the order, leaving me alone with Robert for a few minutes. I heard a gurgling sound.

Horrified, I watched feces come out of Robert's mouth and nose at the same time. In all my hospital experiences I had never seen anything like that. The memory is etched in my mind in a way that cannot be removed.

When the doctors returned, they saw what had happened. There was no time to waste! They inserted a tube through Robert's nose and began to pump. Of course, Robert resisted. Who wouldn't? They had to tie his arms to the rails of the cart he was still on from the echocardiogram. They transported him to 4B and allowed me to accompany him. I remember how different I felt being the mother of a patient with a blocked bowel than I felt as the mother of a patient with a behavioral disorder.

Of course, they had to discontinue the antipsychotic medication because he was having his small intestine pumped. When the doctors had the bowel issue stabilized, they started Robert on an intravenous antipsychotic medication, Abilify, that they administered through the port established for his ECT treatments.

It worked. His psychosis began to improve. I learned later that he could not use the medication given to him in the hospital. The cost of an Abilify injection was too expensive to use as an outpatient. The care he received was excellent. I could visit at any time from 7:00 a.m. to 7:00 p.m. without any restrictions.

He was a real patient. Anyone calling the hospital or sending a card could address it to him and he would receive it. We had many setbacks in the med surgery hospital but there was no problem with his staying there until it was determined appropriate for him to leave. First, he developed pneumonia because he aspirated some of the feces. Then he developed a resistance to the heparin the doctors were using to keep clots from forming in his legs. He was switched to Coumarin, which required additional testing.

Robert developed a high fever that did not subside with treatment. That led the doctors to discover an infection in his port. They had to remove his port and replace it with an alternative venous route for treatments.

They tried moving him to 7B which required less monitoring, but as it turned out he needed the extra monitoring. They brought the emergency equipment to Robert, so he did not have to move again. Another situation that became evident on 7B was that with the close monitoring on 4B, Robert was under constant surveillance by the nursing staff. On 7B, it quickly became clear that Robert required additional monitoring. The hospital provided nursing students to fill that role. He remained in the B building for a total of about six weeks.

He had become acutely psychotic while dealing with the blocked bowel. The physicians were working frantically to try to dislodge the blockage without performing surgery. We were assured it would be better to use a nonsurgical route. Robert was dealing with a nasal tube pumping out his stomach, the symptoms of psychosis, and the enemas (1500 ml) several times a day that were returning only 500 ml of watery stool.

Now and then a resident physician would attempt going through his anus up as far as possible into his colon to manually remove the impacted stool. We had truly descended into Hell. At one point, I lay my head on the pillow next to Robert's distorted face and whispered, "Hang in there, Robert! We have come this far. Don't leave me now. I will not leave you like this!" He did not hear me. Mercifully, his mind had taken him someplace else. He did not remember.

Finally, we were able to get the bowel blockage cleared without surgery. I will never forget the day that the family-practice resident came into the room and cheerfully announced that Robert was ready to be discharged because he was no longer medically acute. I was more than surprised and stuttered, "What do you mean that he is no longer medically acute? He is so psychotic I will not be able to care for him at home!" The doctor replied, "He cannot stay here, he is no longer medically acute." The solution? He was discharged from the med surgery hospital and admitted to the Behavioral Health Hospital when I was not there. I never received discharge papers or instructions. We went back to being behavioral-health patient and family again, with even more of a gap between treatment for the brain and the bowels.

An interesting side story with his bowel was as follows:

Robert had been dealing with psychosis and bowel and bowel and psychosis. He had inherited one of the finest colon experts from his father who had been treated in Indianapolis by a nationally recognized colon expert. Robert's father and Grandmother Lafuze were both polyp formers. For that reason, Robert had his first colonoscopy at forty and because he had polyps, he was placed on a six to seven-year return. Due to the years of the anticholinergic medication, that slows movement through the intestines and causes constipation, Robert's colon was distended.

Janice Comes Onboard

My son-in-law's sister, Janice, came to help me and then stayed to help both Robert and me on a regular basis. She and I worked together when the time came for Robert's scheduled colonoscopy. We followed the instructions for the one-day procedure religiously even though it was difficult. The challenge was coaxing a person who was extremely psychotic to drink all the prep. We had to force Robert to drink the prescribed amount of diluted magnesium citrate solution. Not easy!! We managed despite his bouncing back and forth between I hate you and terms of affection that followed which were strung together like balls on a pop-it-bead necklace.

The worst part was when the gastroenterologist said it was a failed colonoscopy because there was too much fecal matter in Robert's colon. We would have to repeat the process, and this time Robert would need a two-day prep. At this point I called a halt to the situation. It was easy enough for the gastroenterologist to say, but I knew it would be impossible for us to do. I had only been able to do the one-day prep because Janice stayed through the night to help. We explained that there was no way we could do that because Robert would require around-the-clock supervision and the two of us could not provide that. He would have to be hospitalized. That is when the discussion became tense.

We scheduled the repeat and the gastroenterologist said the nurse would call to schedule. The nurse knew what the problems would be and took care of planning for the procedure in a regular hospital setting where the procedure would be performed for a two-day period so that the hospital personnel could administer the solution and clean up after him.

This hospital asked us to state a code word, but it was never used after that. My daughter asked whether the code word was needed because Robert had schizophrenia or because the code word policy applied to all who came into that unit. The nurse assured us that all patients and families needed code words. We gave her Yoko Ono, but Yoko was not needed after that time.

This time the prep was successful. Janice and I applauded ourselves because it took several persons per shift to get Robert to drink the preparation and several persons more per shift over a two-day period to clean up the messes made to accomplish what we did as two people over one day. It helped our morale to think that way.

The insurance paid for all of this. After all, it was a bowel procedure and not a Behavioral Health one. The hospital staff assured us there were many patients who needed to be admitted for the same reason; but this was a regular medical unit rather than a behavioral health one. The colonoscopy worked and we started over with a clean colon.

Robert's Ruined Hand

The lasting memory is what he called, "My ruined hand." During the worst of the blocked bowel episode his right hand was so contracted that he ruptured the farthest tendon on his ring finger that should allow him to straighten that finger out. He used his index finger and his thumb on that hand to do everything.

That is when Erin entered our lives. I was assured that our insurance would cover occupational therapy to help Robert recover the use of his "ruined" right hand. The hitch was that I had to schedule the therapy. I called the number for outpatient OT and finally got a return call. They could schedule a visit later that day. Yay! It was well worth it. Erin (the occupational therapist) was wonderful. She was not only a skilled occupational therapist; she was experienced with working with patients with disabilities. Robert loved her and looked forward to his sessions with her even though they made his hand uncomfortable.

Erin worked his hand in hers, used the paraffin bath, and made him splints. After several sessions, she wanted him to see an arm and shoulder specialist. He was very kind and helpful, but he hesitated to do any surgery. He doubted that it would make any difference in the long run. When I asked him about other patients with contracture, he said that it was not unusual. He had seen patients who had embedded their fingernails into the palms of their hands because they had gripped so tightly. He returned us to Erin's care.

Then Erin suggested another surgeon who had treated some of her other clients with disabilities. We were finally able to schedule an appointment with Dr. Peck. She suggested loosening the tendons on the palm side of Robert's hand. He would still not have full use of his right hand, but it would allow him to work toward being able to straighten his fingers out on that hand.

She did the surgery. We had several follow-up appointments with Erin. She made him some splints. She also suggested that we purchase a paraffin bath for him. When Robert died, we were still in the process of straightening out his fingers. I asked that his left hand cover his right one in the casket. I believe Robert is in Heaven with both his earthly and Heavenly fathers, and Robert has two perfect hands.

Chapter 24

It is a Puzzle That Can Be Solved

We faced even greater challenges with Robert's psychosis. We were able to take him to his ear doctor, psychiatrist, and occupational therapy appointments for his hand. He seemed to be able to "pull himself together" when he was in those situations, but he switched to becoming more and more hostile otherwise. Meeting the fragmented psychiatric system became extremely difficult. The psychiatrist who was treating him in the mental health community center was trying to coordinate a meeting with a neuropsychiatrist.

Another psychiatrist who had presented to my undergraduate class on the Biology of Mental Illness told me about a neuropsychiatrist he worked with who treated patients at St. Vincent Hospital on the north side of Indianapolis. I was able to schedule an appointment for Robert with that neuropsychiatrist who did imaging.

The reason I had such hope was because I was attending Grand Rounds for the Department of Psychiatry and had learned there that imaging was being used to determine what was going on in the brains of patients with dementia. That imaging was on patients old enough to qualify for Medicare because the project was covered by grant money from Medicare. Indiana University has a phenomenal program specializing in Alzheimer's Research. The funding began years ago due to the efforts of a neuropathologist who did seminal studies. That project supports many researchers who study dementia, but Robert was too young to qualify as a patient.

Few patients with Robert's disorder, schizophrenia, live long enough to reach Medicare age. When Robert was diagnosed officially at age 23 or so the average age of death for persons with schizophrenia was 51 years. In the last few years, it has begun to climb a bit. One reason is that there is beginning to be an effort to treat persons with schizophrenia more holistically. Now there is a realization that the need for watching blood pressure, blood sugar, heart rate and other consequences of the psychiatric medications is critical.

I believe the monitoring of the bowel obstructions is lagging. It is recognized that the anticholinergic medications slow down the passage of food through the alimentary canal, so chronic constipation is a recognized outcome. However, it takes longer than the 51-year expected survival, for persons who have schizophrenia, to suffer a totally blocked bowel. Robert was almost 53, and fortunately already in the hospital, when his blocked bowel episode occurred.

Sometimes, in the face of an impending blockage, doctors recommend a surgical procedure to make an opening attached to a bag that needs to be changed frequently. That sounds like a solution. The problem is that a person with an illness who functions well enough to wander off but is too confused and psychotic to manage such a system is only slightly better off than one with a blocked bowel. Even under the watchful care for persons living in group homes the constipating effects of the anticholinergic medications can lead to death due to blocked bowels.

One of my friends who is a psychiatric nurse has a brother with schizophrenia who is in hospice care because his blocked bowel ruptured and the doctors have removed so much of his intestinal tract he faces death due to infections that cannot be medically controlled.

Robert survived because he accepted our stringent care. He was discharged from the med surgery unit following a blocked bowel because he was deemed medically not acute. He was, however, so psychotic that he was admitted to the Behavioral Health unit. He was discharged from that unit three weeks later. The doctors took him to surgery to replace his port which had become infected with a staph infection.

They replaced the port on a Friday afternoon after his ECT in the morning and called me to come and get him during the visiting hours. He came back from surgery after 5:00 p.m., and I was there to pick him up. The doctor had left. The nurse handed me his discharge papers and told me I could take him home. No one read his instructions to me.

Worse yet, the unit kept leaving phone messages stating they had indicated wrong medications in several instances. We found other errors. Even worse, I had to take him back to the emergency room (ER) at the same hospital complex on Saturday morning after he was discharged Friday late afternoon. Although he had left the med surgery unit three weeks earlier, he had developed an impacted bowel that the ER doctor removed by going through his anus and rectum and reaching as far up into his bowel as his arm would go. I watched as the doctor removed four to five pounds of solid stool. Then he took a picture to document what he had just removed.

There is no way to hold that unit accountable because there are no patient or family evaluations except internal ones that patients can choose to fill out if they wish. All of this in the name of confidentiality. Such confidentiality kills.

When we got him home, Robert continued to deteriorate, especially with respect to his brain. We scheduled the brain scan that the neuropsychiatrist finally ordered. When he examined Robert in the office, he stated that he was not sure what a magnetic resonance imaging (MRI) would show, but he said he could rule some conditions out. The images I had seen at Psychiatry Grand Rounds were images using functional magnetic resonance imaging (fMRI) which show blood flow to the areas of the brain.

The fMRI brain scan that captivated me was of a patient old enough to qualify for the study. She could be identified loosely as a dementia patient. However, the scan showed no impairment in the portions of her brain that would allow her to understand the instructions she was given. The only impairment was in her ability to act on those instructions. What captivated me was the explanation that went along with the picture. This woman was not intellectually impaired at all. Her cognitive mind was perfect. However, she could not follow through on commands. She was unable to dress herself. Oh, my gosh, I thought. That is close to what we had with Robert.

He understood every word I said. I know that because I knew exactly what questions to ask and how to ask them. I could interact with him when he was psychotic and get him to respond in a way that let me know his cognitive skills were intact. My frustration was due to his inability to follow through on what he fully understood. That was the same challenge as the patient whose brain scan I had seen at Grand Rounds. When I dressed him, I had to move his body to turn him around. I had to place my hands on his hips and turn him the way he needed to go.

It is a puzzle that can be solved. I know it can; but the research will not be done until we start looking for reasons that the brain of a person leads to the symptoms we see. I have a dream that one day we will not judge a person by the behaviors he or she exhibits. We will understand those behaviors as symptoms of an ill brain. We will not describe a person by generalized illnesses based on symptoms of a brain disorder. Rather we will describe that person's disorder as specific to certain brain regions.

If I could see the future in a crystal ball, I hope that I would see physicians looking at a brain scan of a person who exhibits symptoms of a disorder that would be diagnosed as schizophrenia today. However, the physicians in the future might be saying to each other as they look at the brain scan of that patient, "This person has a lesion here," as the physician points to and names a specific place on the brain scan. "Look, I see another here in a different area and yet another down here." Continuing to gaze into that crystal ball I see experts in treatment from many perspectives such as psychotherapy, medication, laser surgery, and magnetic field exposure, as they work to improve existing treatments and discover new ones. Who knows what kinds of therapies the future may bring?

Chapter 25

I Come to Terms with the Reality of Where We Are in Medical History

I tried tirelessly to take advantage of the opportunity of having Robert on the least amount of anticholinergic medicine as possible. I consulted with a colleague who had never met Robert personally, but who had worked with a neuropsychiatrist who had done some research on schizophrenia. My colleague intervened to get Robert and me an appointment with the neuropsychiatrist. I learned through this experience that a neuropsychiatrist is truly a neurologist.

It is projecting into a future possibility that a neuropsychiatrist will be a part of a marriage between neuroscience, psychology and psychiatry. That day is not here, but I know it will come. When I was a student at IU Bloomington there were cognitive psychologists, but even those were hidden in research labs. All these years later I know how far we have come when I go by the psychology building in Bloomington and read, "The Department of Psychological and Brain Sciences!" Yay!

We began our journey with the neuropsychiatrist with his order for a magnetic resonance imaging (MRI) of Robert's brain. An MRI shows more detailed anatomy of the brain than either an X-ray or CT scan. I had hoped for imaging that included not only the anatomy but also blood flow to the brain.

The first attempt was at an outpatient facility which proved futile because even though they permitted me to hold his hand Robert could not remain still enough in the chamber to keep from moving. It was not that he was uncooperative, he simply could not hold still.

The second attempt was an admission to the hospital where the neuropsychiatrist practiced. They had to reschedule because Robert was too agitated. The third attempt was at the hospital with Robert under sedation. That time they were able to finish the MRI, but the neuropsychiatrist's interpretation of those scans showed no abnormality.

I came to the sad realization that we had pushed the medical system to the limit. The medications that had kept Robert rational for so many years had taken their toll on what had begun as a normal digestive tract. Keeping Robert's best interests at heart, I set a new goal of working with the psychiatrists as they did all within their power to help keep him as rational as possible with the least amount of damage to his bowel. Weekly electroconvulsive therapy (ECT) treatments were an important part of that plan. The wonderful ECT team at the Methodist Hospital continued to support us well, right up to the very day that Robert died.

Chapter 26

Is It Possible to Find Coordinated Treatment for a Brain and a Bowel?

I spent May 2016 through May 2018 trying to find a medication that would work effectively with the psychosis but not damage his bowel. Who could treat both the brain and the bowel? Janice, my son-in-law's sister, (wonderful Janice) had let me know months in advance that she planned to take a vacation with her husband the first week in April. I had made plans with an agency that we had used for my care after I had hip and knee replacements in 2015.

The CEO visited my home and assured me that they would send a person out to do an assessment of our situation so that they could meet our needs. As the time came closer and no one had come, I called to ask about the situation. Finally, I received an email from one of the managers that they would not be able to help us. I was devastated and called; a woman explained their shortage of personnel. She told me they were so sorry, but their faithful few were having to choose between their regular clients because they could not meet all the needs. And then God stepped in, as the Almighty seems to do.

When I need an angel, an angel shows up. In this case the angel was a former student who became a colleague. Codie Kirby had lived with Robert and me many Monday through

Thursday nights when she was a student in Indianapolis. Then she commuted home for the weekends, to be with her husband who was staying at home with their children during the week. Since that time, she had been through a divorce and her ex-husband had the children every other week. Her children had a two-week spring break and she had them the first week. The second week they were to be with their father, and Codie was able to stay with me from Sunday night through the next Monday morning. She told me she wanted to spoil me because I had most of the care of Robert from Saturday to Sunday night and until Monday morning when Janice came and after she left on weekdays at 3:00 p.m. Codie was here that entire week around the clock.

On Friday afternoon (April 7, 2017) we had a meeting when another of my angels, Andrea Turner, was meeting with me with school-related issues. While we were working, Andrea looked up to see Robert standing in feces. He had tried to make it to the bathroom but the medicine that the gastroenterologist had put him on caused him to have explosive bowel movements. It works by holding the stool in the colon until it pulls in enough water to force evacuation. Robert was always meticulous about his bowel habits and made every effort to make it work, but this was a situation he could not make work.

It took all three of us two and a half hours to clean Robert, his clothes, the flooring, and the bathroom. Codie said, "I cannot leave you like this." She got on my computer and found the most appropriate program that sounded as if it could meet both his bowel and brain needs.

Codie and I took Robert to that hospital and admitted him through the emergency room. The psychiatric intake person and the emergency room doctor told us that he would be put in the triage center of the community mental health center where he was usually seen. It sounded ideal. I was able to visit him. There were individual rooms where patients could be monitored. Robert seemed to get along okay, but I was unable to talk with a psychiatrist. The nurses were very nice and helpful, but I had hoped to speak to the psychiatrist about the medications.

On Sunday afternoon (April 9), while I was at the hospital to visit with Robert, I recognized a psychiatrist I knew from committees we had worked on together. She came over to talk with me. She was unaware that she was caring for my son because she did not connect our last names. She came over to talk only because she recognized me. As we talked the conversation changed to how she had cared for Robert. She commented that she had increased his medication.

The next Tuesday (April 11) the hospital called me to come and get Robert. I called Bryce (my son-in-law's nephew) to ask him to stay with us, which he did. In the night Robert became very agitated and banged hard against the door between the back room and my room. We called 911 and the police came. I greeted my new best friend, Lt. White, a Crisis Intervention Team (CIT) officer.

The CIT model was developed in 1988 in Memphis, Tennessee. The goals of CIT are to train law-enforcement officers in the recognition of mental illness, to enhance their verbal crisis de-escalation skills, and to provide more streamlined access to community-based mental health services. The Memphis community soon realized the benefits of this advanced course of training through dramatic declines in injury rates among both citizens and police officers, decreased utilization of the SWAT team to resolve crisis situations, and—when safe and appropriate—the diversion of people with mental illness from incarceration to community-based mental health services. Today, CIT training is available to local police and sheriffs throughout the country. Instructions for persons in need of CIT are to call 911 and ask for a CIT officer.

Chapter 27

We Go Round and Round on a Not So Merry a Merry-Go-Round

Robert calmed down enough to agree to go back to the hospital, so Bryce and I took him in our car. The police led us to the hospital emergency room, and he was readmitted to the triage unit. The next morning (April 12) the behavioral-health specialist at Midtown Triage called me to tell me that Robert had not met criteria and that he would be discharged to the street unless someone picked him up by 10:00 a.m. I told her I was on my way to work at IU East in Richmond and could not be there so she increased the time they would hold him until noon.

To keep from missing work, I called my sisters, Jan and Mary, who picked Robert up at the hospital and brought him to our house. Bryce agreed to meet them there. When Janice and I returned from Richmond, Bryce was holding the fort.

Robert was agitated and began being hostile and aggressive again. This time Bryce and I called 911 and they transported him in the ambulance to the hospital. The positive to come out of that incident was the actions of the CIT. Always when I call 911, I ask for a CIT officer. When the police arrived my new best friend, Officer White, was there first, but police officers kept coming through the front door. I heard each succeeding one coming in ask the officer ahead of him, "Are you CIT?" and received an affirmative response. Each officer was dedicated to assuring there was a CIT officer on site. NAMI Indiana deserves accolades for its sponsorship of such a wonderful, dedicated group of people who train and become CIT officers. They are among the angels who bring God into the room.

The triage unit called me on Thursday (April 13) to come and get Robert. Janice and I picked him up. I stayed with him alone during the night against my better judgment. Let me explain, I was never afraid of him as long as he recognized me as his mother, but when the delusions and hallucinations tormented him enough, I realized he did not recognize me as myself and would attack me as if I were someone or something else tormenting him. He came at me before I could get the door between us closed. He flew into the room. I fell as I staggered backward, hitting my head on the floor. He was on top of me, but I was able to get ahold of his arms and wrap my leg around his legs and talk him down. I lay there with him until he finally calmed down enough to fall asleep. When Janice came on Friday morning (April 14), we were able to get him to the hospital and admit him through the emergency room.

My youngest daughter, Mary, her husband, Steve, and kids, Tom and Kayla, came Saturday (April 15). The hospital sent Robert home Saturday morning because he did not meet criteria. When we tried to admit him again, they informed us they were unable to accept patients because they were under diversion, which meant they were filled.

They said that Methodist Hospital was under diversion also, but Community North Hospital might have beds. Steve drove while Mary sat in the backseat with Robert. We had a difficult time because we had been told to take Robert to the emergency room. The Emergency Room told us to go to Behavioral Health, but Behavioral Health seemed closed. We walked through the door finally and were instructed to ring the buzzer. The woman who came out told us to leave Robert because there were three people ahead of him to be interviewed and each interview would take at least two hours.

We went to eat. Afterward, we sent Tom and Kayla home in Mary's car because she had driven separately from Steve and the two grandchildren. Behavioral Health at that hospital held Robert for evaluation, saying it might be all night, so they would call us in the morning (Easter Sunday, April 16). The next morning as we were headed to church the phone rang. It was Community North saying that Robert did not meet criteria. They had someone ahead of him who needed the last bed they had, so he did not meet criteria. We needed to come immediately, or they would release him to the street.

My daughter, Leanne, went to pick him up and met us at church before the service began. Robert sat through church. At certain points the tears flowed out of his eyes, but he wiped them away and made every effort not to cry. It broke my heart to watch. He was agitated enough to draw the attention of worshippers sitting nearby, but ours is a reconciling church. All are welcome, including people who exhibit symptoms of mental illness. Thank God! We made it through the service and managed to keep Robert calm during lunch.

Mary and Steve agreed to spend the night. I slept downstairs, but we put Robert in his room upstairs at the front of the house. Let me explain that at that time he believed I was not his mother. He had been having delusions that I was a monster who was turning him into a dog. He even said to Mary, "See my paw, a monster is turning my hand into a paw!" and pointed to his arm.

Steve slept in the bedroom upstairs that was at the back of the house, just beyond the stairway. We set up a mattress for Mary at the top of the stairs so she could intercede if Robert tried to come down the stairs. She was afraid he might stumble down the stairs in his confusion. She heard him go to the bathroom next to his bedroom. Then before she could catch him, he flew past her and down the stairs and straight for me in my bed. I screamed for help. Mary was trying to take a video, to document this psychotic episode, but she had to put the phone down to try to pull Robert's hands from around my neck. We were able to get his arms immobilized and stop him. I held onto his arms so my daughter could call 911. She asked for a CIT officer, who came quickly. The emergency response personnel said this was an Immediate Detention (ID) and that meant a 72-hour hold. They took Robert to the hospital in an ambulance.

Monday morning (April 17), they called from triage telling Janice and me to come and pick Robert up or they would release him to the street because he did not meet criteria. What had happened? He was on a 72-hour hold. We were sadly misinformed. It really meant the hospital could hold him up to 72 hours, but of course, they could determine that he did not meet criteria before that. That is what they did.

I asked who had made the decision to release him. I was told it was the psychiatrist in consultation with Robert's psychiatrist. How could that be? The police had to pry him off me. I was on the phone to the psychiatrist who has been faithful to Robert and our family for over twenty years, off-and-on. I asked, "How can this be? How could he not meet criteria when he demonstrates being that psychotic?" The doctor replied, "He does not meet criteria because we have no beds!"

That Monday (still April 17) when I called Robert's psychiatrist, he suggested we come by his office so the nurse could give Robert an injection to help calm him. We took him to the psychiatrist at the Community Mental Health Center, who took time out of his very busy and full schedule to meet with us, only to hear him say he had no further suggestions. I know that made him sad. Our hands were tied.

Then Janice and I decided to go with Robert to the Methodist Hospital Emergency Room. It is the best I have ever frequented. We decided I would go in as the victim of his attack. I hated doing it, but we told them he had a diagnosis of schizophrenia and needed to be evaluated.

Here is how that played out. They separated Robert and me. I was now an official victim of domestic violence. I was examined thoroughly, including an X-ray. Robert was left alone in the Methodist Hospital Emergency waiting room, which caused me some concern. Janice did the best she could to keep an eye on him. When she needed to leave, Robert had no one to watch him. When it came time to evaluate him, he had left the area. This fact was reported to me and I was cautioned to be careful when I got home because these men find ways to get back at their domestic partners. If I had not been so worried about Robert, I could have gotten a good laugh over that one.

I tried to explain that was the least of my worries. If Robert got outside the hospital he would likely be picked up by the police and end up in jail. I was frantic. From inside the Methodist Emergency Room examining room I called 911. I explained where I was and what had happened. I must credit the 911 operator. I had hung up the phone after I called, and she called back. She asked whether I had contacted Methodist Hospital Security. I did not know how, so she established a three-way conversation.

Just as security was about to send out alerts for Robert, the nurse practitioner came back in and said he had reappeared. He told them he got lost. Evidently, he had gone to find some-one to give him money to try to buy a Coke out of the Coke machine. When he came back in, he had a Coke and a piece of pizza. What a charmer that son of mine can be! To this day we have no idea where he obtained that piece of pizza. They discharged me after taking CT scans of my head and neck. And they kept Robert for evaluation.

We received a call from the hospital the next morning (April 18) saying we needed to come to sign some paperwork that Robert met criteria and would be admitted. We had mixed feelings about that. Yay! He met criteria, but we were concerned he would be back on the Behavioral Health unit on the eighth floor. 8C is wonderful and a Godsend for patients who need the kind of therapy the unit offers. But Robert's illness was too severe. The good news is that they kept a very, very close eye on his colon (bowel movements), and that, along with the fact that he was accepted at a time in which there were few beds, was enough to keep us going. We have learned to look for the blessings in each day, so those sufficed.

The person who evaluated Robert found a spot on 8C. It was literally an answer to prayer. It gave us time to plan while Robert was in a safe place. Robert was started on a new antipsychotic regimen and released to a rehabilitation center. I took Robert's arm-splint in because the occupational therapist who treated him in what seemed to be the same hospital could not treat him as an inpatient. One learns to choose carefully when there are so many questions to ask and points to be made.

The occupational therapist who made the splint assured me there was an occupational therapist who served that unit. I should take the splint in and she would instruct the staff on how to put it on each night so that his hand could be stretched out. It was a plan. I took the splint in, but who knows what happened to it after that? It did not make it to the rehab facility where it was supposed to go. I know, because I was there to check what came with him from the Behavioral Health unit and the splint was not there. I talked to nurses from every shift who knew nothing about it, including the night nurse who told me she had not only not put it on him, she had never seen it nor received any communication regarding it.

When I contacted the "Mental Health Consultant" who was responsible for coordinating the affairs of the unit, she knew nothing about it and had her supervisor contact me. The supervisor said that none of the staff had any knowledge of where the splint was. I asked for the name and number of her superior, whom I contacted. He had a staffer contact me claiming that the hospital was not responsible for lost personal items. I knew it was a lost cause. I assured her that I was not about assigning blame but was about solving problems. This item was not a personal item. It was, in fact, a part of Robert's therapy. She listened but told me she could do nothing to help me.

When I contacted Occupational Therapy, they told me that the department could make a new splint if they had a doctor's order for it. What doctor would write such an order? The quickest resource was the facility where Robert was staying for nursing care and rehab. I asked the manager whether there was a doctor who could write the order. He assured me there was, and he could decide whether Robert needed to be transported and have the splint made.

The afterhours occupational therapy facilitator said she could give the manager the number for the order to be faxed, how he could schedule the time and the occupational therapist most available could make the splint, but they could not provide someone to stay with Robert in the waiting room. But the manager said they could provide a staff member to come with Robert—and the problem was solved.

How can a facility not responsible in anyway come together so easily to solve a problem at hand? Part of my answer is that it is not subject to the same stigma-producing and restrictive confidentiality burdens as a behavioral health unit would have. It is a general nursing and rehabilitation unit. Most of their patients are either post-surgery or other non-surgery patients requiring rehabilitation services. They are used to solving challenges of persons with multiple needs. Surely, we can provide as well for those who have been diagnosed with the brain-based disorders that we call mental illnesses.

A related issue is the funding source for behavioral-health services. Many families are encouraged to drop private insurance and/or Medicare in favor of Medicaid because that is how many agencies are reimbursed for behavioral-health services. Although I was told Robert's care could be covered by Medicaid, I was blessed to be full-time employed at the time of Robert's death. I persisted to keep him covered by my private insurance and his father's Medicare, and finally we added Medicaid as tertiary. I envision a day when decreased stigma and improved therapies will diversify funding sources for medical care and living costs for persons affected directly by mental illnesses.

Chapter 28

Our Journey South Begins

Robert was admitted to a rehabilitation center south of downtown Indianapolis. It was an excellent facility where he received physical, occupational, and speech therapy. The goal was to get him physically stronger, cognitively more alert, and have the occupational therapist stretch his right hand. Because of his tendency to wander, he had to wear an alarm trigger on his ankle. Unfortunately, the alarm trigger interfered when we had him outside the facility for some doctors' visits and other therapy sessions.

During his stay at the rehab center, Robert became so despondent that he was admitted to 8C at the Methodist Hospital on a Thursday. The psychiatrist had planned for him to remain on 8C until the following Monday morning when he would be discharged from 8C and admitted to 8B. Her plan was for the hospitalist to look for a way to treat both his brain and his bowel issues together. This was the psychiatrist who had urged me at least a year earlier to undertake guardianship of Robert.

On Monday morning I received a call from the behavioral-health counselor that Robert was released from 8C and I could pick him up or they would provide transportation back to the rehab center. I was in shock. What had happened to the plan? I called the new director of Behavioral Health and had to leave a voice message. He called me back the next day and talked with me for more than an hour. He fully agreed that persons with psychoses had brain-based issues. Finally, it became clear that he was probing. The behavioral-health counselor had told me that all that they needed to do was inform me as Robert's guardian that the decision had been made to send him back to the rehab facility. My objection to that was that the behavioral-health counselor was, in fact, making a medical decision. The call of the behavioral-health director was to determine whether the psychiatrist had made the decision, or the behavioral-health counselor had. When the behavioral-health director finally put it that way, the answer was easy. The behavioral-health counselor told me she had made the decision and the psychiatrist had gone along with it.

The Behavioral Health director had probed until his reason for calling was answered. After that determination my ability to communicate with the C unit of the hospital ended. The behavioral health-counselor, another administrator, his secretary and the behavioral-health director all refused my calls. I was particularly sorry that the other administrator, who was also a friend, shut me out. And I feel certain that the reason was fear of a lawsuit. However, I will always be grateful to that psychiatrist for making sure the Electroconvulsive Therapy (ECT) group knew that I was Robert's guardian.

Let me explain further. Several days later I received a call from the ECT Coordinator. Robert had been signing for his own treatment. Now that they knew I was his legal guardian I became responsible for his treatment. The ECT Coordinator told me I would need to come in person to sign a form approving the ECT treatment prescribed by the Community Mental Health Center psychiatrist. When I told her Robert now had an Indiana University (IU) Health psychiatrist, I did not have to come in person. I was able to call in and give approval over the phone if two registered nurse witnesses were on the line.

The last two ECTs that Robert received were administered in the cardiology unit under the jurisdiction of their anesthesiologists. I felt that the move to the main building of Methodist

Hospital was a positive step. Rather than being conducted in the behavioral-health wing, future ECTs would be held in the main hospital. The psychiatrists were the physicians who would administer the treatment, but the anesthesiologists required me to be available by phone when they called because I was Robert's legal guardian. The calls worked like a charm the two times that Robert went to ECT under this new plan.

Having Robert go to ECT from the rehab facility south of downtown had its advantages and its drawbacks. The facility provided transportation but could not often provide someone to stay with Robert during the treatment. That was perfectly understandable and acceptable because my family and I could not imagine how the facility did such a wonderful job of caring for their patients with such a small staff. However, it led to some very interesting challenges. Usually, it worked well because Janice could meet Robert at the hospital and wait with him until the transportation provider returned to pick him up. One day the rehab facility changed the ECT transportation to a Tuesday, even though the ECT unit was not even open on Tuesday. The man in charge of transportation let Robert off, thinking Janice would be there to meet him and left Robert roaming the halls of the very large Methodist Hospital. Someone recognized Robert and knew the ECT department was closed on Tuesday. The person who found Robert took him to the entrance where the receptionist watched him until the rehab driver came back to pick him up. All was well. Why do I share this story? I share it because, somehow, we have been blessed to have angels in every shape and form watch over us.

One Friday when I took Robert to ECT, I heard a patient in the waiting room call out, "You were my teacher!" She had been a student in my Biology of Mental Illness class. She continued, "Little did I know then that I would become a patient." She told me that she had learned about ECT in my class. She had resisted her father's telling her that ECT was barbaric. She remembered a lecture by Dr. Schmetzer, a well-known expert in ECT. Dr. Schmetzer had explained that ECT was so safe it was the method of choice for women who were pregnant because all activity took place in the brain and did not affect the baby at all. She thanked me for the class and all that she had learned that was helping her at that time.

Finding a New Psychiatrist

I was frantic. I needed to find a psychiatrist affiliated with Indiana University (IU) Health where the rest of Robert's medical needs were met. While Robert was in the rehab facility, we were forced to use the psychiatrist for that facility. He visited on his own schedule; therefore, I never met him or had a chance to talk to him. Every bit of information about his treatment choices for Robert came through the facility nurses from his notes. I was frustrated because there was no choice about Robert's care while he was in that facility. However, it did give me an opportunity to think about his care when he was released.

The Community Mental Health Center that had served him well for several years was not a part of Indiana University (IU) Health. The plan was to move Robert to an independent-living situation with another client or two and around-the-clock care. I could no longer care for him by myself around the clock. Although the ECT psychiatrists were a part of IU Health, I could not pursue my search there because they did not see patients outside the hospital. The neuroscience center used residents in psychiatry, but there were not enough staff psychiatrists to supervise them. The other community mental health centers would not take more patients with schizophrenia from Center Township (downtown Indianapolis). Indiana University Health has four facilities around the outskirts of the city. Only one psychiatrist in all those four hospitals was taking new patients.

I considered Robert in crisis. He was suffering hallucinations most of the time. When it was his bowel, it was a crisis, but his brain disease was not considered a crisis. It was August, and the first available appointment with a psychiatrist was January 15. The scheduler was so very nice. I tried my best to stay calm through all the Behavioral Health talk. The final blow was as follows: The nice lady told me that she would call me back in the event of a cancellation. I assured her that if I missed the call, I would see her effort as a missed call and call her back. I asked what number would show up on my screen. The reply: "Oh, this is a behavioral health unit so it will show a blocked number. You won't be able to call it back. It is a fake number."

Suddenly, I thought of Mom (my grandmother). She had a "Hush, hush, we do not talk about this disease" (cancer). We hid it under a bushel basket. This is like leprosy used to be before we knew about Hansen's bacillus. Dear God! How can we move forward if we cannot even have a conversation about a brain that is causing these symptoms? I choked up. The lump in my throat crowded out my voice box and triggered a switch that formed tears in my eyes that rolled down my cheeks.

I struggled to let the "nice lady" on the phone know that we were still connected. It was certainly not her fault that we have a system that treats a "broken brain" differently from how it treats a broken hand or a broken bowel. It is not her fault that this is a hush, hush disease. Oh, how I wish I could assign the blame to her and bring closure! I long for closure, but I remember the lesson I taught our children so well when they were young that they remind me in their maturity, "We are not here to assign blame. We are here to solve problems!"

The nice lady on the phone waited for me to calm down so that I could speak. Of course, she waited. She dealt with emotional people all day. Oh, if only all our culture could learn from her. If only those who dealt with broken hands and broken bowels and broken hearts could slow down to listen and wait for those dealing with the emotional components of those disorders to calm and speak.

The nice lady assured me she would call back to let me know whether the psychiatrist might have an opening before January or whether there was a psychiatrist at another site with an earlier available opening. She kept her word. I answered the cell phone I had cradled close to my body so I would not miss the call. She was amazed and allowed it to show in her voice. None of the psychiatrists in all three other facilities under that group were taking new patients. I had already been rejected by the other groups outside of our township because Robert's diagnosis was schizophrenia and we lived in the inner city (Center Township). I wondered what I would do if the discharge date from the rehab facility left a gap between the availability of a psychiatrist to write the necessary prescriptions for Robert until January.

The good news was that I found a wonderful psychiatrist in the IU Health system who would accept Robert as a returning patient because he had treated Robert before when he was a psychiatrist with the ECT team. It helped that Robert came to him as a private patient who had Anthem as his primary insurance, Medicare as secondary, and Medicaid tertiary. His office staff were always kind and supportive. Crystal, the nurse who worked closely with him, was especially helpful.

Chapter 29

Transition: We Lived Betwixt and Between

The trauma of the blocked bowel took its toll on Robert.

The Brain is a Complex Organ

The effect on Robert's brain was striking. He short-circuited back to before the accident. It was unsettling to take him to the car and hear him say, "This isn't our car. Where is our car?" Then I heard him describe a car we drove when he was a teenager. When he was in rehab and I sometimes took him to his house on Paca Street, he did not remember it as his house. He asked, "Will we be in trouble for breaking into someone else's house?" These incidents taught me well the power of psychosis. I learned to respect even more the complexity of the brain, especially a brain when it is not well.

The Blocked Bowel Trauma Affected Us All

The trauma of the blocked bowel left us all changed. Robert emerged from the psychosis that resulted from the combination of having to take him off the anticholinergic medication abruptly and the trauma induced by the repeated enemas. He recovered slowly and was in and out of the hospital frequently. When he was in the hospital, the doctors changed the medications often. When he was out of the hospital the psychiatrist tweaked the medicines. Thank goodness for the ECT treatments. The major side effect of ECT is short-term memory loss, but his improvement was worth every bit.

Realizing that I would not be able to care for him after he left rehab, I began to shop around our neighborhood for a house I might buy so that Robert could live with one or two other people who had serious mental illnesses with around-the-clock staff Medicaid would provide. The existing small "group homes" were more than a mile away and that was too far for me to monitor Robert's care.

Ralph had invested in stock from the time he was an undergraduate student at Purdue. He worked summers and over breaks as a surveyor. He was able to pay for school and to invest. When we moved to Hagerstown, he met a man named Mark Hale who served as pastor of a church and was an investment consultant for Edward Jones in a nearby community. They did well together, and Ralph's portfolio thrived, even after Ralph's death in February of 2012. In 2017, it was the money in that portfolio that I had intended to use to buy a house at the end of Paca Street. I was sorely disappointed when the house was sold to someone else.

Chapter 30

Dad's Still Taking Care of Us

When I shared my disappointment of losing out on the purchase of the house down the street, my oldest daughter, Jeannette, said, "Mom, John and I have been looking at properties large enough for us, his mother and a nephew. We found one that had a large house, a barn and a mother-in-law house on ten acres we loved, but we do not have enough money to qualify without Dad's help."

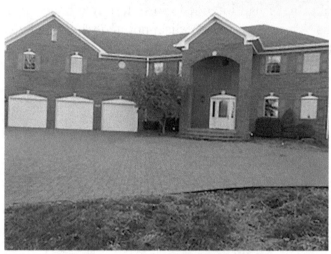

The "Big House" with acreage and the
barn. It also had a guest house.

Mark, of course, resisted my taking the money out of the account until he heard the details about the property. I remember his exact comment, "It seems that the stars are aligning here."

When we were sure that the deal was a possibility, I took Robert to see the mother-in-law house. He had become weary of the rehab center and was ready to go home, which his brain had "tricked" him to believe was still in Hagerstown, even though it had been at least a decade after any of us had lived there.

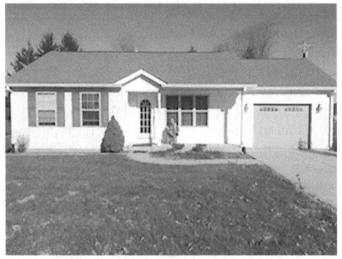

Robert on the porch of his new home

The mother-in-law house was a two-bedroom house with a large garage and a kitchen, living and dining area. Robert had been withdrawn on the trip down from the rehab center. We went in and got to the bedroom that became his bedroom. I asked whether he liked it. He answered, "Oh yes! This is really nice." It had been a long time since I had heard him respond with so much enthusiasm. "Would you like to live here?" His nod was enthusiastic. It was the happiest I had seen him for weeks. On the way back to the rehab facility, Robert asked, "Mom, how am I going to pay to live there?" I told him about the money Ralph had left. "Your dad is still taking care of us, isn't he Robert?" Robert replied, "He sure is!"

That was the end of October in 2017. The move-in date was set for November 20. Robert and I crossed the days off on a calendar he kept by his bed in the rehab center. We called this new house "Robert's House." It was the second house to bear his name. Living in what was now Robert's House was a stabilizing factor. Although he was extremely psychotic, our visits to the hospital were limited to emergency room visits and ECT.

It took several months and persistence from Leanne and me to finally find a wonderful caregiver, Lisa Hampton, who provided services through Medicaid from midnight until 8:00 a.m. We were constantly tweaking medications to treat the brain and avoid extreme issues with the bowel. Working through multiple issues with the social security and Medicaid system brought a number of people into Robert's small house.

The wonderful psychiatrist through IU Health worked with us to adjust Robert's medications appropriately. With his consent, we were able to add large doses of niacin and CBD oil, which had a calming effect. The most successful part of Robert's treatment continued to be ECT. He was now receiving those once a week on Fridays, and he enjoyed improved cognitive function at least through Monday. Only once did the doctor try extending the interval to two weeks, but the symptoms warranted returning to once weekly.

The medications clearly caused unfortunate side effects. Robert was confused and withdrawn. The ECT treatments brought him out of that withdrawal but unfortunately the effects lasted only a few days. While there were still challenges, Robert was the happiest we had seen him. At Christmas 2018, Robert so enjoyed the family and festivities.

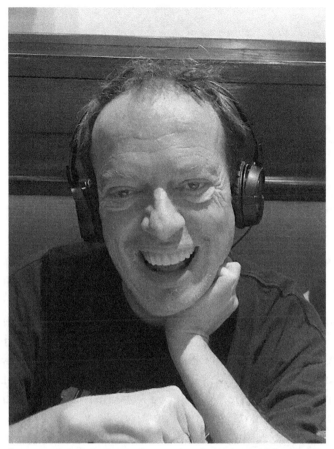

The joy on Robert's face shows that in spite of his challenges, living in his own home gave him moments of great happiness.

Chapter 31

Death (March 1, 2019)

The morning of March 1, 2019 started out like most Friday mornings. My daughter, Leanne, who is a physical therapist, came to Robert's house south of Greenwood to treat me with a special therapy, myofascial release (MFR). Lisa got Robert ready for Janice to take him to IU Methodist for his ECT. He needed to be fasting from midnight on. It was an easy one for Robert. We put a pink tie on the refrigerator door to remind him that he would need to be fasting after midnight. No worries. He loved the ECT sessions and looked forward to them. "Oh Mom, they help so much with the voices! Nothing else helps as much!" We all looked forward to Robert's ECT.

Leanne came and left. Janice returned home with Robert. They had stopped at McDonald's for his standard kid's happy meal—a plain hamburger, French fries, and Coke and a small frozen custard for dessert. He ate the "ice cream" first and took a few bites of hamburger and one or two French fries. Janice had given him his meds and I was giving him the CBD oil. As I gave him his CBD oil, I quickly checked his mouth to be certain he had swallowed his food, and I put the oil under his tongue.

During the time he ate, Janice shared that he had a nice conversation about the rock group, Rush, with the psychiatrist while waiting for the anesthesiologist. She had also shared that a patient across the hall was hollering that she did not like ECT and wanted to refuse it. Robert was calm and ready. He told one of the nurses, "You look nice today." On the drive home he gave Janice that same compliment. It was a good day.

When Janice got back to the house, she told me that once Robert was lying down, she would switch cars by putting one in Jeannette's garage and the other in the garage at Robert's House. The problem with that plan was that Jeannette had had a total hip replacement the day before (February 28) and her physical therapist's vehicle was blocking the garage door in front of the "Big House." After Robert went to his bedroom, I called the administrative assistant of Indiana University East's school of Natural Science and Mathematics (NSM) to schedule an appointment with the interim dean. I was talking to her when Janice went to check on a thud from Robert's room. She came back to tell me Robert was having a seizure or something. I cried out, "Oh, my gosh, Robert is having a seizure!" The administrative assistant said, "Hang up the phone and take care of Robert!"

Janice and I ran to the bedroom. By that time Robert's face and neck were a dusty pink. I wondered whether he was aspirating and called out, "Robert breathe, please breathe," as I was trying to do the Heimlich maneuver. For one instant, I saw Robert's head turn toward me, just as his father had done when he heard my voice the day he died. Then Robert was dead weight. Janice managed to get 911 to report that we needed help. She gave the address, and the wonderful 911 operator assured us that help was on the way. Then he said, "In the meantime roll Robert over on his back and start compressions right over his breastbone." We finally managed to get Robert turned over and I started the compressions, but I was going too fast, so Janice took over. The 911 operator said, "That's better," and Janice and I managed a laugh. I kept begging Robert to breathe. "Please breathe for me, Robert. Just breathe."

The chaplain for the Bargersville Police Department arrived, then the police, and a number of others piled into Robert's

House. Finally, the paramedics arrived, saying they had gone to the "Big House" first. When they came into Robert's bedroom, they suggested they needed more room to work and invited Janice and me to wait in the living room. That is when I met the chaplain and all of the police contingency, including the deputy sheriff.

My son-in-law's mother came over because all of the emergency crew had gone to the "Big House" first. She wondered whether something had happened with Jeannette. Janice told her that the concern was a situation with Robert, but she did not go into detail.

The person in charge explained the procedure to me. "We have not had a spontaneous breath or heartbeat so far. We will work on Robert for a half hour. We will stop every 10 minutes to see whether he takes a breath on his own or we detect a heartbeat. We will inform you of our results and continue until 30 minutes have passed. At that point we will discontinue our efforts and call the coroner." I asked whether we could transport him to the hospital so that my daughters could help me decide what to do. The answer was "no," and I nodded. The procedure began. After 30 minutes the nice man called the coroner.

The chaplain suggested that I call Crown Hill Funeral Home in Indianapolis. When I called, I told them the coroner was on the way and requested that they send a hearse to take Robert to the funeral home. The woman replied that if it was a coroner's case, I would need to come in person with identification to sign papers before they could do that. I decided to come in the next day. The chaplain kept shaking his head no, but she was insistent. I found out later that he also worked with the Indianapolis Metropolitan Police Department. The only time they had a coroner's case was if there was suspected foul play. We were in a different county, so the procedures were different from those in Indianapolis.

The coroner came and assured me on the way to Robert's room that he would explain why the funeral home would pick Robert up, but he had to go to Robert's room first to complete his official duties as the coroner. When the coroner came out of Robert's room, he asked Janice and me what had happened. He also asked for a list of Robert's medications and whether I wanted a picture of Robert's ID. Janice took the picture. He took Robert's medicine bottles and ruled that there was no need for an autopsy. He was documenting the cause of death as a pulmonary embolism because it fit those criteria of events, our account, and the medicines Robert was taking. At that point all of the police and deputy sheriff left. The examiner gave me his card and left.

The coroner explained that he had an "in" with the funeral home and they were on their way. The chaplain stayed until one of the pastors from our church in Indianapolis arrived. The pastor stayed until my daughter, Leanne, came. The coroner stayed until the funeral home took Robert with them.

I called the ECT coordinator and was surprised when she answered the phone because it was after hours. I told her Robert would not be there for his next ECT because he had just died. A few hours later, I received a call from the psychiatrist who had treated him that morning. He thanked me for taking his call. "I hated bothering you at this time, but when the nurse coordinator told me, I couldn't believe it. Robert was doing so well this morning. We talked about his music and he was in such a good mood. Do you mind letting me know when you set the time for the visitation?" Not only did he come but also the entire ECT team including Laurie, the nurse coordinator who had just retired. A former member of the ECT team who was serving as Robert's psychiatrist at the time of his death also came.

My need for closure was overwhelming. Every other parent I knew who had buried a child, and there were many, understood that need. I remember when my mother said, "How wrong it is for a parent to have to bury a child." Thankfully, she was spared. She was 101 when she died and all three of us were still alive.

We planned for Robert's celebration of life for Friday, March 8, with the visitation from 3:00 until 7:00 and the service at 7:00. The funeral home planned for the family to have from 2:00 until 3:00 at the church to set up for the service and spend time with Robert. There were several, including one of Robert's most faithful psychiatrists, who wanted to attend in person but could not. I assured all who could not attend in person that they would be with us in spirit. And they were.

Chapter 32

Celebrating Robert's Life

At the memorial service for Robert, his sisters and I gave witness to Robert's courage. His sister Leanne wrote the following:

> There are people in this world who have struggles beyond comprehension but shine a light so bright for us. Mom has always said that Robert is our biggest teacher. For a long time, I wasn't sure exactly what that meant. Today, I would like to try to put our lessons from Robert's life into words.
>
> **COMPASSION:**
>
> While Robert allowed us to be a witness to his vulnerability and strength, we learned compassion. In school, I witnessed Robert sometimes being the target of practical jokes or teasing. This was hurtful for me, but it made me consciously decide to try to be nice to others, especially those who are not like me. I, in return, hope that others will show me compassion when I am in need. At

age 53, I am still practicing compassion, grace, and patience with others and myself!

DISCOMFORT:

We are creatures who like to stay away from discomfort, go the other way, ignore or look away from others who are struggling. Robert taught us to go into the discomfort. A couple of years ago, Robert had a major medical crisis and was taken off his psychiatric medications cold turkey. Our family thought maybe Robert didn't need all the medications.

We were very wrong. There were some very intense times watching and holding space for Robert when he was clearly psychotic. At times, I thought my heart would break from the intensity of watching Robert go into this hell. But we could not run away from the intensity and we could not leave him in the dark, frightening hell where he would go sometimes. We just were surviving— especially mom—who never gave up on him.

By going through the discomfort and the total darkness of those times, Robert and our family were also ushered into the light. He was doing so well the past few months and overall the past 15 months when he moved to Greenwood. I have learned that if you can hold on through the darkness, in comes the light. We learned to sit with others in discomfort. To create space to witness the pain, struggles, and suffering of others.

TEAM:

We have learned what TEAM looks like and feels like. Mom has pointed out that we would not have survived without our team. Looking back, our team started with Robert's first psychotic break. I remember being a teenager—so unaware of the journey we were preparing for. At times, wondering if Robert would be better off in heaven than here on earth. These are thoughts and feelings I am not proud of—but they were there. (By the way, compassion also is needed for oneself.)

We were with the pastoral staff at First United Methodist in Hagerstown, and they prayed for us.

Our team has added more and more members over the years, including a strong support at our current church—here at North. Robert was able to come into services for a while and participate after his last hospitalization. He loved singing familiar hymns and he would always say the Lord's Prayer even when he was not feeling well or participating as much.

We have had wonderful caregivers who have stepped up to the plate. A special thank you to Eileen Huber, Irma Boyett (who stayed with Robert overnight when mom was hospitalized), Lisa Hampton, and Janice Wilkins, who stayed with us during some of the most difficult times in the past three years.

I grew up in a family focused on team even before Robert got sick. After Robert's death it occurred to me that my parents co-parented— which was not as common as it is today. Fathers worked and moms took care of the house and children. My dad did the laundry, washed dishes, went to the grocery store and sometimes would take us to school if we missed the bus.

I feel like dad said to my mom last Friday, "You have done such a great job with Robert these past seven years, let me take care of him now."

Robert, we love you and will miss you so much. Our hearts are breaking but we are excited that God has taken you into His care. Saturday, I pictured God receiving Robert into His loving arms and cleansing him. Taking his brain and cleansing it, so he is whole!

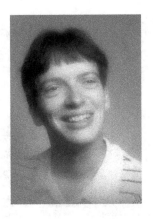

Memorial Sermon for Robert Lafuze
Reverend Darren Cushman Wood
March 8, 2019

I met Robert before coming to North. I met him at NIFS where he walked the track with his headphones on. Later, as I got to know him I learned that the music he loved to listen to was a lot of the same music I grew up with.

I was especially blessed by Robert a couple of summers ago when he was living in the facility on the south side. His room was sparse and so I assigned our summer seminary intern to create a poster of musicians and album covers of the kind of music Robert liked. She was in her early twenties and had no idea what she was doing. When we gave him the poster it was a delight to listen to Robert educating her about classic rock. I am sure that knowledge will stay with her the rest of her ministry and will serve her well! (Continued)

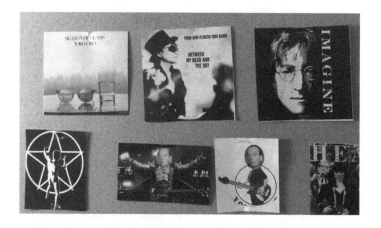

(Pastor Darren's Sermon continues here.)

In honor of Robert and in keeping with his good musical sensibilities, I am basing this sermon on a quote from a Yoko Ono song.

What we celebrate today is that Robert was touched. From the very beginning, he was touched by God's grace. That touch was more fundamental, more lasting than anything else that had touched him. Even through the darkest moments, God continued to hold him. God had touched him with love and gentleness, and in turn Robert touched us with his smile.

In the Christian tradition, there is a connection between the rites at the beginning and at the end of life. In the baptism of infants, we celebrate that God touches children and calls them beloved children of grace. And at the end of life in the funeral ritual, we affirm that God welcomes the child, at any age, into the fullness of eternity where we are fully known by God as we truly are. What defines us is not our diagnosis but our baptism. In baptism, we put on Christ and so in Christ we are clothed with glory through the power of his resurrection, the power of eternal love. Thus, as Paul's words to the Romans rings true for us: Whether we live or die we are the Lord's.

The bond which you shared with Robert continues on. This is the bond of the Spirit that connects our souls with those who live on in the eternal love of God. Robert once asked which is closer: Heaven or Florida. The answer is clear: Heaven is closer because of the common touch of the Spirit. God touches us with comfort and hope in our loss through this bond.

Out of our loss comes new understanding of what we go through in life. We realize the ways God was at work with Robert that changed us forever. (Pastor Darren closed Robert's service with the first verse of "Hymn of Promise.")

Chapter 33

"Then You Will Know the Truth and the Truth Will Set You Free."

(John 8:32, Christian Jubilee Bible)

I believe in absolute truth. However, I am very cautious about deciding and declaring exactly what constitutes that truth. Tracing what is true is tricky. Using rest stations along the journey as final "stops" can do anything but set us free.

I implore you, the reader, to consider this section very carefully. I have personal opinions about the need for gun laws, but those are not a part of my reason for writing about the relationship between mental illness and acts of violence. My sole purpose in this account is to share what Robert taught me and my family.

Persons Who Have Mental Illness Are Rarely Violent

Dr. Alan Leshner wrote an article published in the August 16, 2019 edition of *Science* titled "Stop Blaming Mental Illness." His article included a finding supported by the Council for Behavioral Health that people with mental illness are responsible for less than 4% of all violent crimes. Such a statement shines light on the fact that persons with diagnoses of psychosis such as schizophrenia, bipolar illness, and severe depression are more likely to be victims of violent crimes than perpetrators.

In another article published in *Time* magazine on August 19, 2019, authors Dr. Jessica Gold and Dr. Megan Ranney address the same topic. Dr. Gold is a professor of psychiatry at Washington University in St. Louis, Missouri. Dr. Ranney is a professor of emergency medicine at Brown University in Providence, Rhode Island. The title of their article is "It's Not About Linking Gun Violence and Mental Illness." The message in their article is the same as Dr. Leshner's: there is no factual link between mental illness and violence against others.

Both articles are so very true and well worth your taking the time to read in their entirety. The *Time* magazine article details the stigmatizing effects of linking mental illness and violence against others that made the article painful for me both as a neuroscientist and as a family member to read. However, it is that stigmatizing factor that prompts me to continue with lessons from Robert. I believe it is the fact that we continue to label brain-based illnesses "behavioral" that prevents early detection and early intervention. Dr. Tom Insel, former director of the National Institute of Mental Health, explained the importance of these facts eloquently in a presentation at the California Institute of Technology in 2013.

I heard a person with a diagnosis of schizophrenia say once that schizophrenia is a subtle disorder that robs a person of how to know what is true and what is not true. However, we in the general public think of schizophrenia as anything but subtle. In those rare instances when the hallucinations and delusions of psychosis take control, the outcome can be violent.

A Psychotic Break from Reality Can Change a Person

Robert taught us that it is possible to have no memory of actions during a psychotic break from reality. I was fortunate because even with the incredible strength he could generate during an adrenaline-fed psychotic frenzy, I could break his hold. I could wrap his small body in my arms and anchor him between my legs.

I have read newspaper accounts of teenagers or young adults who have committed crimes. Some have had mothers and/or fathers show up for their court hearings. I remember reading about one young man whose mother rubbed his back and neck as the judge was making his sentence longer because he showed no remorse for what he had done. "Show remorse," I said aloud to an empty room as I read the account. His brain is ill. He may be terrified and trying not to show it. My heart went out to that mother because he may not have been small enough for her to restrain. She knew what Robert taught us so well that her son and mine were vulnerable and in need of love and reassurance.

I pray for a day when we will be able to live in a world that is focused on solutions rather than on assigning blame. It will be a day when we end criminalizing brain-based disorders such as mental illness and addictions. On that day we shall provide humane care for those persons who are most vulnerable themselves, especially when they are not safe for others to be around. We are not ready yet as a society to understand what Robert was able to teach our family well. When a person suffers the kind of illness he had, no matter how good that person is, there may be times when he or she is not safe to be around. That situation calls for a safe place that provides protective, humane care. But we are not "there" yet. We need research to provide more effective treatments and even perhaps a prevention or cure.

Robert was able to teach our family that it is possible for a person who is kind, loving, and protective of others to become hurtful when under the influence of psychotic illness. Our first advantage was that we were so very much blessed by the fact that when Robert had his initial break from reality, Ralph acted immediately to seek help that involved three medical doctors who saw that he was hospitalized the same day.

The second advantage we had was that Robert had amazing insight into his illness. Once the medications worked, he knew he was ill and realized the importance of the medications.

Accounts of other families have made us aware of a lack of such insight in some situations.

A final advantage we had was that Robert was a "Pinmaker." He was small enough for me to be able to restrain him long enough for assistants to intervene. I take responsibility for seeking ways to reduce the anticholinergic load after his blocked bowel to find imaging that simply is not available now.

Society is Focused on Seeking Justice for the Victims of Violence

Understandably, our hearts ache for those victims who have suffered unjustly. It is right that we bestow honor on those who help these victims. However, I envision a day that we will also seek understanding and compassion for those persons who are acting in response to brain-based hallucinations and delusions. My long-range prayer is for Robert's and my family's story to be part of a transformation that includes early detection, early intervention, and possibly even a cure for these brain-based disorders we call mental illnesses.

Why I Wrote This Book

I ask myself, why have I written this book? My immediate answer clearly is to share our family's journey with our remarkable son and brother. In the words of his "little sister," Robert has truly taught us the most important lessons of life.

My second reason is to pay tribute to every kind, caring, compassionate, and competent person we have met along the way of this journey. I write with confidence that the professional people who have held us in their hands and hearts are dedicated to those of us who are personally affected by these brain-based disorders that the world calls mental illnesses. My goal in this writing is to draw attention to the fact that these dedicated professionals are bound in a web spun by a spider that traps them in a system that is fragmented. These dedicated people are like carefully honed puzzle pieces with neither a complete picture nor frame to go by.

The third reason is to mark our family's place on a continuum. As Dr. Dunlop explained to Robert, the brain disease he had has been traced back to ancient times. World-wide, people with schizophrenia and many other forms of dementia were "housed" in asylums. More recently in this country, state hospitals served that role until the emergence of antipsychotic medications and other forms of treatment permitted people with such diagnoses to come into the mainstream of our society. Robert and our family were on the leading edge of that transition.

I remember the blackouts, the nightmares that became "daymares" because they did not go away after Robert woke up. I remember my own "daymares" because I was fully conscious and rational, dealing with a system that made no sense.

It was painful for me to read *This Stranger, My Son* by Louise Wilson. Her son, Tony, and his family represent the previous era on the timeline. The Wilson family entered about twenty years (a generation) before our family. I read her account of the psychiatrist's incorrect explanation that Tony came into the world with a mind that was a blank slate and they, his parents, were his problem. They had caused his schizophrenia. She was the major cause, he said, but her husband was also to blame. The psychiatrist closed the conversation by telling them that Tony and they would be better off to be separated.

Tony knew that his parents loved him. He realized his painful vulnerability when he was rational. He loved his family, but he could not control lashing out at them. Louise Wilson never gave up hope that one day her son would be able to come home permanently to live with them.

She ended the book with the following paragraph:

Under all the fear and anger, he has faith in our love. When his mind is clear, and perhaps even in clouded hours, he knows our love will last. It will be there always; it is there now, waiting for the joyous day when Tony may come home to us all again. (Wilson 223)

140

How grateful I am that Robert and our family came a generation later on the timeline than the Wilson family. We had the advantage of better medications, even with the bad side effects. We also had the advantage of more effective treatments, such as improved ECT. Except for the times that he was in the hospital or rehab, our family was able to know the joy of having Robert live with us. We did not have to wait for him to come home to us all again.

Mary's Poem

"Which is farther: Florida or Heaven?", the young boy asked his mom.
Puzzled, she replied, "I can't answer that, my son."
As she watched him grow she shared his pain,
his troubles broke her heart.
Why was life so cruel to him, this boy so sweet, so smart?
And as she thought of the road ahead, and all that he'd been through,
she remembered his question of long ago, and cried because she knew
Florida was so far away — the fun, the sun, the joy.
Life was tears and fears and woe for her precious little boy!
But she felt a sense of peace, as she smiled in her despair.
Heaven is much, much closer, you see, and she knew he'd make it there.

Three Tributes to a Man Whose Life Made a Difference

The following are three of the tributes from the Crown Hill Cemetery webpage. I have removed the names. The first is not from Rocky. It is from another elementary school friend.

It is with a sad heart that I hear this news. I met Robert in kindergarten and was a big brother to him throughout our elementary years until he moved away. Since I was a bigger kid. I made sure no one picked on my brother. I took the job very seriously and with great love. I ran into Robert and his mother a few years ago at Ponderosa in Greenfield and was very happy he and his mother both remembered me. Great memories with an awesome kid. God Bless and fond memories, my brother.

I am so sorry for your loss. I have never forgotten how Robert came to my defense when we were in elementary school. Some older boys were picking on me and he stepped in and distracted them from me. He had a good heart.

Joan, as a mother, I am so sorry for your loss. Though I did not know your son, you shared your story with me years ago, when I was a student and first struggling with my own child with mental illness. I never told you, but this was a profound moment that I have never forgotten. This has helped me understand so many things over the years, so your son helped people far beyond what he might ever have known. I thank you and thank your son.

References

Adler, R. & Ross, J. (1953). Acorn in the Meadow. Frank Music Corp.

Cavinder, F. B. (April 1962). *The Indianapolis Star*.

Chambers, R. A. (2018). *The 2 × 4 Model*. New York: Routledge.

Chambers, R. A., & Wallingford, S. C. (2017). On mourning and recovery: Integrating stages of grief and change toward a neuroscience-based model of attachment adaptation in addiction treatment. *Psychodynamic Psychiatry. 45* (4): 451-474.

Gold, J., & Ranney, M. (August 19, 2019). It's not about linking gun violence and mental illness. *Time. 194*, 34.

Lafuze, J. E. (February 10, 1980). *Star Magazine*.

Leshner, A. I. (August 16, 2019). Stop blaming mental illness. *Science. 365*, 623.

Sleeth, N. (1986). Hymn of Promise. Hope Publishing Company.

Wilson, L. (1969). *This Stranger, My Son*. New York: A Signet Book.

Additional Information

Google Tom Insel Ted Talks to hear a 17-minute presentation in which Dr. Insel states steps toward early detection and early intervention that are much needed in treating the brain-based disorders we call mental illness.

Mental Health America (MHA) website: www.mhanational.org

National Alliance on Mental Illness (NAMI) website: www.nami.org

About the Author

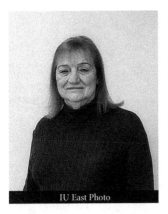

IU East Photo

Joan Esterline Lafuze, Ph.D., is a Systems Medical Physiologist and has been a Professor of Biology at Indiana University East since 1987. She was appointed Assistant Professor part-time and Research Associate at the Indiana University School of Medicine in 1981. Dr. Lafuze received her Ph.D. in Physiology at Indiana University School of Medicine in 1981 and taught there until she accepted her current teaching appointment at Indiana University East. Dr. Lafuze conducted fulltime research in Pediatric Hematology/Oncology from 1981 until 1987 and has continued to collaborate at the Indiana University School of Medicine. She and her family have been active in The National Alliance on Mental Illness (NAMI) Indiana since its inception. Dr. Lafuze has become fascinated with the tremendous strides made in basic science research related to those disorders that have traditionally been considered "behaviorally and socially" based. Her involvement in teaching and translational neuroscience research provides a "springboard" for a multidisciplinary approach to understanding these illnesses and the complexities of treatment strategies.

CPSIA information can be obtained
at www.ICGtesting.com
Printed in the USA
BVHW042329191020
591090BV00012B/55